CatchFire

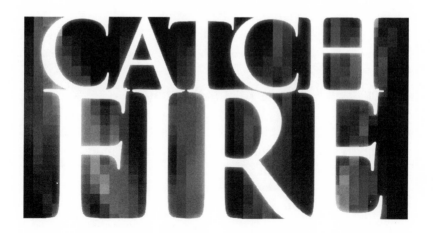

CATCH FIRE

*A 7-Step Program to Ignite Energy,
Defuse Stress, and Power Boost
Your Performance*

PETER MCLAUGHLIN
WITH PETER McLAUGHLIN, JR.

A MCLAUGHLIN COMPANY PUBLICATION

A McLaughlin Company Publication
Originally published by the Ballantine Publishing Group

Copyright ©1998 by Peter McLaughlin

Visit our website at: www.petermclaughlin.com

Library of Congress Cataloging-in-Publication Date
McLaughlin, Peter J.
       CatchFire: a seven-step program to ignite energy, defuse
       stress, and power boost your performance /
       Peter McLaughlin

               p.   cm.
       Includes bibliographical references.

       1. Success - Psychological aspects. 2. Mind and body.
       3. Stress management. 4. Success in business. I. Title.

BF637.S8M3644   1988
646.7—dc21

Manufactured in the United States of America.

First Edition: January 1998

10 9 8 7 6 5

"Compared to what we ought to be, we are only half-awake. Our fires are dampened, our drafts are checked, we are making use of only a small part of our mental and physical resources."

—William James

"The tongue of flame . . . the volcano . . . these are the most affecting symbols of what man should be. . . . A mass of fire reaching from earth upward into heaven, this is the sign of the robust, united, burning, radiant soul."

—Ralph Waldo Emerson

CONTENTS

ACKNOWLEDGMENTS

This book is a product of fifteen years of research and seminars, first with Jim Loehr, a world-renowned sports psychologist, and now at McLaughlin Company, where I share the research and writing with a team of experts that includes my son Peter.

I'd like to acknowledge my mentors and friends who have been major influences in my career. The wit and genius of Marshall McLuhan, the late media guru, and my colleague Edward Maginnis, S.J., of Regis University, have had a tremendous impact on my thinking and life. I want to thank Bill Daniels and John Saeman for giving me my first opportunity to present seminars to the people at Daniels & Associates.

Peter and I benefited greatly from the creative advice of many colleagues and friends who helped by reading chapters, offering criticism, or discussing ideas over a bottle of wine. These include Ken Petri, M.D., Steven Forness, Ed.D., T. George Harris, Doug Scott, Christina Hathaway, Michael J. Little, Thomas Tierney, Barry Triller, Steve Gesing, Barry Elson, Steve Baldwin, Vinnie Sestito, Brian Keating, David Pemberton, Rob Gleser, M.D., and Art Stone. Our agent Peter Ginsberg has been a great source of enthusiasm and counsel.

Additionally, we're grateful to the many people who offered encouragement and support, including Shannon Walsh, Wendy Nevalls, John Atencio, Carrie Ochitwa, Steve Narans, Carol Petri, Maureen Brooks, Marcia Rothenberg, Randy Hickernell, Regis Malloy, Jeff Griffiths, Andrea Thornbury, Leif and Pat Smith, Peggy Tighe, Mary Lee Ryan, Janie Volkert, Jennifer McLaughlin, John McLaughlin, and Anne McLaughlin.

Finally, I'd like to thank the staff at Ballantine Publishing Group (which published the original edition of *CatchFire*), especially Susan Randol, Linda Grey, Clare Ferraro, Leona Nevler, Ellen Archer, and Shannon Atlas.

CatchFire

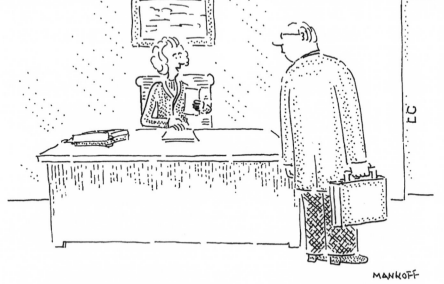

"Sir, the following paradigm shifts occurred while you were out."

INTRODUCTION

Reenergizing Yourself to Thrive in a Changing World

The new world of work is shaping up as a far scarier place . . . riskier, less dependable, more anxiety-provoking.   —Jack Patterson, *Business Week*

"You're juggling ten things at once, rushing from meeting to meeting, phone call to phone call, one thirty-second hallway conversation to another, scribbling notes back and forth on typed memos. You're constantly nudging initiatives forward, moving from issue to issue, all the time trying to stay focused."

Sound hectic? It's just another day at the office for Barry Elson, the Executive Vice President of Operations at Atlanta-based Cox Communications, one of the nation's biggest cable and communications companies. In addition to staving off new competition from the phone companies, negotiating with government officials, and orchestrating the smooth integration of a recently acquired company, Elson is helping Cox dive into *six* new businesses. "We're pressed to get into these businesses very quickly—in about an eighteen-month period—which is a killer series of tasks, particularly when they are brand-new businesses," says Elson. "We don't have anyone who knows about them, so we have to hire outside expertise, which means we have to absorb new people into our culture." Combined with the task of trying to keep up with a frantic pace of technological innovation, Elson and his cohorts at Cox face a dizzying degree of change, complexity, and uncertainty.

On an individual level, Elson says, the experience of going to work has become a challenging ordeal. Every day he walks through the office door, he faces a rigorous test of his stamina, composure, and ability to think under fire. And while he thrives on the opportunities and excitement of his job, he says that—without question—the personal demands have never been greater. "I've been doing this for twenty-seven years, and this is certainly the most stressful period I've gone through," says Elson. "There's a hellacious amount to get done. There are new demands on people. And the pressure is not going to stop."

I've worked with Cox for over a decade, giving presentations to divisions across the country to help all levels of their workforce prosper in a competitive, rapidly changing environment. I didn't work with them to revamp their customer service policy, restructure their work processes, or revitalize their strategic planning. Rather, I helped the people at Cox—as I've helped people in hundreds of companies across the continent—reenergize *themselves.* That is, my seven-step CatchFire program taught them how to use the remarkable breakthroughs in mind/body science to maximize their energy, focus, and productivity at work. From attitudes and thinking patterns to diet and exercise to relaxation and humor, I detailed the most valuable concepts and tools that mentally and physiologically prepare people to thrive in a demanding world.

At Cox and at companies around the globe, the high-pressure work environment is forcing people to expand their idea of what it takes to be a top performer at work. Knowledge and expertise aren't enough anymore. Working productively, making good decisions, and maintaining cooperative relationships with clients and coworkers all require a more basic capacity: the ability to stay energized, focused, and fun in the midst of chaos.

Unfortunately, most people respond to today's demands in ways that undermine their ability to maintain a focused and energized state. Instead of upgrading their lifestyle to accommodate a tougher schedule—the way you would upgrade your computer's memory to handle a powerful new software program—they fall into a pattern of detrimental habits that sabotages their productivity. If you have the lifestyle of an average American, this means you eat too much, exercise too little, and don't take enough time to relax your body and mind. It means you probably spend much of your workday feeling tense. And it means that very likely, you aren't having enough fun. Like an overloaded computer, people with poor attitudes and lifestyle habits work slowly, break down frequently, and constantly operate on the verge of crashing.

By following the steps of the CatchFire program, however, you can develop the energy and emotional control that enable you to work at your best. Enlisting the support of scientific strategies to maximize the functioning of your body and brain, you can more adroitly handle adversity, solve problems, and inject a spirit of fun into your work. Following these practical steps helps you take a whole new approach to your job—seeing your challenges with fresh eyes, as a Buddhist would say—and totally transforms your results.

The Brave New World of Business

While few people have a "to do" list as formidable as Barry Elson's at Cox, everyone has it tougher these days. Whether you're an executive vice president or a frontline employee, whether your company is a global software corporation or a local coffee shop, you have to grapple with greater demands and intensified pressures. Longer hours, increased responsibilities, constant change, heightened competition, an accelerated pace of business, concerns about job security—the difficulties of life on the job today have assumed daunting proportions. They've made it especially challenging to maintain the physical energy, emotional calm, and mental concentration needed to work creatively and productively. Listening to people talk about how they're feeling at work often reminds me of a comment by the comedian Steven Wright: "You know when you're sitting on a chair, and you lean back so you're just on two legs, and then you lean too far and you almost fall over, but just at the last second you catch yourself? That's how I feel all the time."

Underlying the changes and the widespread uncertainty in today's world of work is the fact that we are in transition to a whole new economy—a whole new world, even. Marshall McLuhan, the communications expert and author of *Understanding Media* and *The Medium Is the Massage*, was one of the first to appreciate the vast dimensions of the transformation. As far back as the 1960s, he pointed out how the industrial age was giving way to the information age, how the world was assuming the character of a "global village," and how changes in technology were beginning to profoundly alter our lives. ("We create our tools, and thereafter they recreate us" is how he put it.)

One of the outstanding features of this transformation, and one that drives a great deal of the anxiety in the world, is that change itself has changed. That is, changes in technology and in society now take place at an unprecedented pace, a pace inconceivable in earlier eras of history. E-mail, faxes, cellular phones, cable networks, the Internet, feverish advances in computer software and hardware—these agents alter the education, health care, entertainment, government, and communication systems of people around the world. And perhaps most dramatically, they alter the world of business.

100 Miles per Hour

Throughout the interviews I conducted for this book, people invariably told me that this relentless pace of change was a major force in making their jobs more complex and challenging. Many other trends—new technology, globalization, greater competition, and new management systems—contribute to making work an intense experience. To get a concrete sense of the personal demands created by such a complex environment, consider three brief profiles of life on the job:

• "As much as everything is changing right now, it's very difficult to be on top of everything at any point in time," says Paul Hoffman, formerly Vice President of Worldwide Communications at Oracle Corporation and now Vice President of Worldwide Sales at Documentum Inc. As Hoffman helps Documentum develop their global sales organization, he says the nature of his work is remarkably different from what it was in the past: "It used to be that you went to school to get trained, you got trained in a certain specialty area, you did a certain job for a few years, and all of a sudden you were kind of a guru. You could go on automatic pilot, and go through the rest of your career just doing what you're used to doing." But as Hoffman says, "that's certainly no longer the case." One of the biggest challenges he faces is the never-ending need to update his knowledge and skills. "You have to constantly learn, you have to constantly reeducate yourself in order to be even competent in your job, much less a leader," he says. The process definitely keeps business exciting. But on the downside, Hoffman says, such a schedule never lets you stop to catch your breath: "You never 'get there.' There is no finish line. You're constantly challenged to stay on top of things—or you get left behind."

• William Merriken, Senior Vice President at Polo Retail Corporation, says Polo's management team has completely realigned the way they run their business to create more customers and offer superior service. On the management level, their strategy entails an aggressive push to open new stores around the world. On an individual sales level, their plans require more energetic and dedicated sales efforts. "Everything was more casual ten years ago," says Merriken. "Compared to our service level today, we were fairly lackadaisical." The revamped sales training includes a far more active approach. "There's a big focus on performance and ways to educate someone to enhance contact with the customer," says Merriken. "It's proactive rather than reactive. Everyone has goals about contacting customers and accumulating new ones." And despite the emphasis on measurable performance, when you're on the floor, you have to look like you're out for a stroll in the park (it is Polo, after all): "If it doesn't feel relaxed, it detracts from our environment. Everything should appear to be easy and comfortable on the surface, but underneath, it's go-go-go."

• Marty Paradise, General Manager of Microsoft's Southeast Region, says that despite Microsoft's dominant position in many markets and their all-time-high stock price, people constantly feel the pressure. "We're always pushing the envelope," says Paradise, "asking ourselves, 'How can we do things better, faster, and cheaper? How can we do more for our customers?' We don't take our success for granted—it takes a lot to be a leader in this industry." The dogged competition and towering expectations that surround Microsoft lead to demanding workloads, a breakneck pace, and a bewildering array of tasks. "My people are going a hundred miles an hour and are expected to generate great business results, create value for their customers, and work with their teammates," Paradise says. "And at the same time, I'm saying, 'Keep your skills sharp, keep up with all our strategies and our competitor's strategies, and be proactive in managing your career at the same time.' "

Playoff Season

All told, recent transformations make business in the information age like being in the playoffs—the competition, speed, and pressure have assumed a heightened intensity. In terms of your daily experience, the changes amount to this: you have to work smarter, react quicker, think brighter, and perform better than you ever have.

That doesn't mean you can't have a good time. Like the playoffs, the current environment offers more stimulating challenges and invites you to stretch your abilities to new heights. So while you're facing more rigorous demands, you're facing them in an atmosphere that is a hell of a lot more exciting than in times past.

As Marty Paradise says about his challenging job, "I love it. I'm having a lot of fun." Corporate structures of old promised most of their people stability and security. But they also promised them boringly industrious lives; they blunted their imagination, stifled their creativity, and relieved them of their native spirit of curiosity. Unshackled from the dull, rigid, and painfully narrow-minded hierarchies of the industrial age, people at every level have a greater chance to personally contribute and a greater freedom from anally retentive bureaucracies.

But for many people, the aggregated pressure and change tip the balance from "exhilarating" to "stressful." Day after day of juggling ten things at once, constantly pushing to meet deadlines, and putting in long hours behind a desk or on the road is proving physically and emotionally draining for a large segment of the population. A recent poll conducted by Northwestern National Life Insurance Company showed the effects of this environment: over 70 percent of the working population agreed that "job stress caused frequent health problems and made them less productive." Another survey by *Industry Week* magazine revealed that 68 percent of Americans say that they "don't have fun at work." Many people have been pushed past the point where increased demands create better performance; instead, their jobs are making them unhealthy, discouraged, angry, and unproductive.

To thrive in today's business environment, however, such a state is entirely unacceptable. Put bluntly, you don't have a chance to succeed if you're sluggish, timid, resentful, and tired. In a constantly evolving environment, the race goes to the quick, to the flexible, to the resourceful, and to those who can generate a sense of excitement about their work. And since the reigning forces of chaos and upheaval don't appear to be abdicating anytime soon, you have to concentrate on the other side of the equation and change *yourself*. As the historian Walter Lippmann wrote of living in the chaotic twentieth century, "We must find within ourselves the certainty which the external world has lost."

The challenges loom large. By adopting new habits and attitudes, however, you can boost your energy, resilience, and—

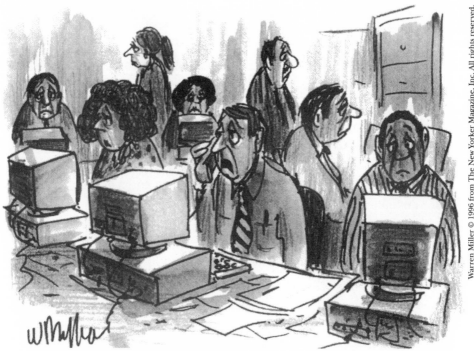

"No, the computers are up. We're down."

adversity be damned—your sense of humor, and use these forces to help you prosper in the new world of business.

Lighting Your Fire

Fortunately, advances in the demands of work in recent years have been paralleled by another set of advances: the virtual explosion of research on strategies to help your body and brain function at their best. The discoveries stem from the fields of psychology and physiology—the studies of the human mind and body, respectively—as well as studies such as psychobiology and biochemistry, which illuminate the intimate connection between the two. For convenience, I'll call this field of study mind/body science.

Mind/body science studies how thoughts and feelings affect us on a physiological level, as well as how physiological changes manifest themselves in moods and mental capacities. Put more simply, mind/body science is based on the idea that every emotion you feel has tangible biological underpinnings. For instance, the emotion of anger is associated with a rapid heart rate, accelerated breathing, high blood pressure, and a relatively high level of the "stress" hormones epinephrine and norepinephrine (also known as adrenaline and noradrenaline) in your system. The feeling of relaxation, on the other hand, corresponds to a reduced heart rate, low blood pressure, decreased muscle tension, and a biochemical profile consisting of relatively low levels of "stress" hormones and relatively higher levels of the "calming" neurochemical serotonin. The complexity of the research is mind-boggling and the amount to learn is formidable; but with greater and greater precision, researchers can describe how your feelings literally change the chemical composition of your body, and how changes in your biochemistry influence how you feel and behave.

The reason this is vital to your performance at work is that certain states of mind—or, put differently, certain states of biochemistry—facilitate clear thinking, confidence, enthusiasm, and productivity, while other states can lead to stale thinking, poor judgment, and bungled performances. Have you ever gotten angry in a big meeting? In addition to the surges in heart rate and "stress" hormones, the emotion changes the way your brain processes information, which cripples your ability to think clearly or creatively. The usual result is that you act irrationally and create friction with those around you. Feeling discouraged leads to a similar disruption in your ability to make good decisions and maintain high levels of productivity. When you get discouraged, your entire biochemistry becomes depressed. Your system is depleted of the chemicals that induce enthusiasm and determination; your brain remembers past failures and expects the worst; and you work sluggishly and unimaginatively, or simply give up.

Contrast that with having a positive state of mind. When you're energized, focused, and fun, you spark a physiological state that predisposes you to work persistently and productively. Possessed of such a mind-set, you confidently pursue your goals in the face of pressure. You assault tough assignments with creativity and verve. And you improvise your way through difficult problems the way the great saxophonist Branford Marsalis improvises his way through a solo. The difference in your mind-set—whether you're angry, pessimistic, or energized—has a substantial effect on your performance.

Further, as scientific research shows, you can train yourself to create a stress-resistant, energetic, focused state of mind. This idea is a relatively recent one. For most of the history of psychology and medicine, authorities have directed their studies to pathology and illness. They have investigated the ways people become depressed or sick, and have experimented with treatments to get them back to normal. More recently, many researchers turned toward a different emphasis. Instead of concentrating on illness, these researchers are exploring the causes of health, happiness, and top performance. Greatly aided by information on the mind/body connection, they are identifying thinking habits and lifestyles that enable people to improve their health, increase their energy, and enhance their ability to excel in their pursuits.

The results of these studies are particularly important to businesspeople attempting to succeed in a high-pressure environment. Most people consistently engage in habits—such as letting negative moods dictate their actions, eating a diet loaded with sugar and fat, or allowing themselves to become overly serious—that prevent them from working productively and becoming successful. But by changing these patterns you can enhance all facets of your performance. For example, if you regularly work out, eat right, and maintain optimistic self-talk, you can stay positive and productive even when your department is being reorganized or your team members display an agonizing lack of common sense. Or again, if you strategically plan a routine that consists of going for a five-minute walk, eating an apple, and doing a deep-breathing exercise at 3:00 P.M., you can resurrect yourself from the typical afternoon slump and work productively for your remaining hours at the office—ending the day with a bang instead of a whimper.

Building CatchFire

My experience in this field began when I studied and collaborated with renowned sport psychologist Dr. James Loehr. Loehr was one of the first psychologists to systematically explore the mental side of professional athletics. He didn't teach people the mechanics of a forehand or jump shot; he focused on how they could optimize their performance by developing more control over their energy and emotions. From extensive work with world-class athletes such as Jim Courier, Pete Sampras, Monica Seles, and Olympic gold medalist Dan Jansen, Loehr developed a comprehensive Toughness Training model that has proven effective in helping athletes and executives achieve top levels of performance.

Since working with Loehr, I've continued to study the leading authorities in mind/body science who are researching everything from stress to prayer to humor (yes, they actually study these topics, often with fascinating results), and formulating the best techniques to help people live healthier, more productive lives. Over the last twelve years I've presented these techniques to a wide variety of organizations, and supported company-wide initiatives to help people adopt stress-busting, energy-enhancing habits. And I've developed a seven-step program that incorporates the most useful and practical of these techniques for people in business.

In my research for this book, I conducted interviews with hundreds of businesspeople (including CEOs, managers, and front-line employees) across the continent to see and hear how they practiced various habits—from working out at lunch to taking relaxing vacations to incorporating humor in their workday—that helped them maintain a positive mind-set and improve their productivity. And to get an even better understanding of the most practical, valuable strategies, I commissioned an independent research company to conduct a Professional Workforce Survey investigating the importance of these habits and mind-sets to people's ability to perform at work. In the survey, which was completed by 1,020 people from the United States and Canada, we asked detailed questions about people's habits, attitudes, and lifestyles, as well as their levels of energy, stress, and perfor-mance on the job. As expected, the results demonstrated a clear, often dramatic correlation between positive, healthful habits and high energy, low stress, a positive mind-set, and better on-the-job productivity.

As scientific experts, hundreds of interviews with professionals, and a comprehensive survey attest, the CatchFire program works. Putting these steps into action will create the surging energy levels and enthusiasm that enable you to triumph over whatever problems are thrown at you. As Taoists say, they help you "step on the path" or begin the journey to greater health and prosperity.

A couple of examples illustrate the kind of results the program can produce. I spoke recently with David Nevin, an account representative for Resource Net International, at one of the company's sales conferences. Having gone through the CatchFire seminar a year before, Nevin said that the experience had spurred major improvements in his performance at work. Before the seminar, he told me, he had been struggling in a difficult new sales position. He regularly felt exhausted from long, hectic days at the office. His high-pressure job was taking a negative toll on his health.

By adopting some of the CatchFire principles, however, Nevin turned his life around. Revamping his diet and exercise habits, and making time in his busy schedule to relax and refocus, he jump-started his energy level and rekindled his determination. His renewed vigor inspired a sharp upturn in his sales and made him one of the company's top salespeople (as Larry Stillman, Senior Vice President at Resource Net, says, "Nevin achieved one of the highest levels of growth at the company"). While part of his increased productivity stemmed from an improvement in his knowledge and sales skills, Nevin attributes most of his success to the revitalized spirit that came from adopting a positive lifestyle.

William Slavin, Vice President of the Western Region at IBM Global Services, made a similarly impressive transformation. I met Slavin several years ago when I led a seminar for his division at Peat Marwick. While impressed with the principles of the program, Slavin initially didn't make any personal changes in what he describes as an "unhealthy lifestyle." Even though he subsidized health club memberships for his entire division at Peat Marwick, he never made it to the club to work out himself. "I always thought that health stuff was for other people," he said.

Too many years of a rigorous work schedule and inadequate health habits, however, finally caught up with him. On a trip to a client site, Slavin collapsed. He was rushed to the emergency room, where the doctor discovered he had a bleeding ulcer. Lying on a hospital bed for three days while he recovered, he reassessed the way he was living his life.

The event compelled Slavin to change the way he managed stress, health, and life balance. Incorporating elements of the program into his life, he started an exercise routine. He began to pay more attention to what he ate and drank. He shifted his work patterns to a schedule that enabled him to get adequate sleep at night. And he made a firm commitment to reconnect with friends and establish a social network that had been missing from his life.

The results of these changes have been dramatic, Slavin says, improving both his performance at work and quality of life. It's not that he has set lower sights at work. On the contrary, his challenges at IBM are more difficult than ever, and he still pushes to be the best in his intensely competitive industry. But now, Slavin takes a more intelligent approach to his tasks, balancing the pressures of his job with a lifestyle that allows him to work more effectively, think more creatively, and better enjoy his life. "I have more energy and a more positive mental attitude," Slavin says. "I'm more persuasive with clients, I get more done each day, and I'm better able to deal with a high-growth, high-pressure business. Taking such an approach is a competitive advantage. I'm convinced of it."

Upgrading Your Resources

The goal of the program is not to help you "reduce" stress in the sense that you learn how to eliminate the pressure of the outside world. For some driven overachievers, dropping some commitments, on or off the job, may be a good idea. (If you find that you dine regularly at the wheel of your car, mistake the names of your family and friends, and drop exhaustedly into your bed at night praying that you'll be able to make it through another day, take it as a hint to lighten your load. "Simplify, simplify, simplify," as Henry David Thoreau advised.) But for most people, significantly decreasing workloads and stress is not an option, barring drastic changes in your employment situation or lifestyle. With today's demanding jobs, you can't simply eliminate outside pressures any more than you can prevent the rain from falling.

Rather than cutting your potential sources of stress, adopting positive changes will bolster, revitalize, and inspire you to thrive in the midst of your challenges. Dr. Robert Thayer of Long Beach State University in California—a renowned researcher on energy, tension, and mood—states this idea in a slightly different way. Thayer says that tension arises when your perceived demands exceed your perceived resources. That is, if the perceived demand of completing a major proposal by Friday outweighs your perceived resources of energy and creativity, or giving a presentation to senior management requires a level of confidence that you don't possess, the result is a feeling of stress. By this formulation, making positive changes in your attitude and lifestyle increases your inner resources. Upgrading your health habits and learning techniques to stay calm under fire endow you with the capacity to approach high-pressure situations with confidence and energy, using such adversity to propel yourself forward rather than hold you back.

To make the program as clear and useful as possible, I've arranged it into seven steps. Some of the steps actually have several components, but they all represent a change in your attitude or lifestyle that will create more energy and positive emotion at work. It's not mandatory to follow the steps in order, or to completely master one before you learn about and implement others. In fact, the different steps complement and reinforce each other. But changes in lifestyle and attitude can be difficult to make. Usually, it's not the failure to understand a new behavior that prevents its successful implementation—following an exercise program, for example—but the failure to consistently practice what you know you should do. To help address this difficulty, I've put them in a sequence that makes the changes as easy and effective as possible.

After discussing the overall CatchFire model for top performance, I introduce Step 1, which teaches you how to develop your self-awareness and control your attitude. The next three steps involve improving the way you treat your body, showing you how to eat, exercise, and rest to achieve high energy levels and positive moods. With biological systems functioning optimally, Steps 5 and 6 teach you how to approach your job with a mentality of challenge and a spirit of fun. Finally, Step 7 offers suggestions on concrete changes in your physical office environment to support the previous steps and maximize your health, energy, and productivity at work.

The program works on several levels. Physically, the steps help you improve your health and energy so you can make it through even the longest, hardest, and most stressful days. Mentally, they articulate specific strategies about how to power your brain to help you think with greater clarity and creativity. And emotionally, they give you tools that allow you to exercise a sense of control in the midst of chaos, retaining your cool and poise when the pressure is on. By following the steps you can effect lifelong positive changes—not just reducing tension, but having more fun at work and learning to relish the challenges your career presents.

The Seven Steps to Top Performance

The key to thriving in the tumultuous conditions of today's business climate is the ability to manage your energy and emotions—or more precisely, the ability to cultivate and maintain the state of mind in which you attend to your work with peak levels of enthusiasm and focus. While you might not usually consider this a business skill, few things have a greater impact on your performance at work. "Being an educated person is no longer adequate," Peter Drucker explains in the *Harvard Business Review*. "I think we probably have to leap right over the search for objective criteria and get into the subjective—what I call 'competencies.' Do you really like pressure? Can you be steady when things are rough and confused?"

Of course, you have to know your business, and have a proficient command of whatever communication skills, selling techniques, or marketing strategies you need to do your job. But today's hurricane conditions have added a new emotional facet to work, and beyond knowing the technical ins and outs of your company and your market, you have to know how to keep yourself in a positive, productive mood. Once you've mastered your state of mind, you've created the most potent force in your arsenal, against which no obstacle can stand.

The state of mind in which you work most creatively and productively—what I call the *energy zone*—is characterized by six key elements: energy, confidence, calmness, flexibility, focus, and fun.

In the energy zone, you are able to tap the latent genius that allows you to confidently, smoothly handle even the most intimidating obstacles. At its best, it is an almost mystical experience, akin to what Taoists call *wu wei*, which literally means "without doing, causing, or making." But practically speaking, *wu wei* means gracefully and almost effortlessly solving problems and producing results. The energy zone characterizes the emotional state in which you feel in control, fully present at your job, and engaged in your activities with top levels of energy and mental alertness. It also describes the disposition in which you enjoy your work even as you diligently labor to achieve tough goals.

How do you enter the energy zone? Basically, it involves monitoring your mind-set and actively cultivating a discipline of positive lifestyle habits. By following the seven steps of the program below, you change your psychology and physiology in a way that enables you to consistently work in this energized, focused, and fun state of mind.

STEP 1: MASTERING YOUR MIND
The first step of the CatchFire program involves staying attuned to your energy level and emotional state. With the pressure and change that define today's world of work, this skill of self-awareness assumes a vital role in consistently performing well.

Unless you maintain a somewhat vigilant awareness of your

"Twang! Zip! Thud! Lucky for you, Wilson, that I'm a civilized businessman."

mind-set, you can become caught up in the hectic stream of events. Often, you lose your sense of calm, confidence, and presence, and work yourself into a mental state of anger or tension that detracts from your ability to perform. Many times, this can mean the difference between a good meeting and a poor one, a great presentation and a mediocre one, a successful sales call and a failed one. Unfortunately, many people go through half their workdays uptight, discouraged, or emotionally withdrawn without even recognizing their mind-set or the detrimental effect it's having on their productivity.

Developing your self-awareness, or constantly looking at yourself and your situation with fresh eyes, plays a crucial part in approaching your challenges with all your energy, talent, and genius.

STEP 2: EATING FOR PERFORMANCE

Step 2 involves upgrading your eating habits to support top levels of energy and productivity. Generally, a good diet provides your body and brain with the high-octane fuel it needs to run most efficiently. But your diet is actually more than just a fuel source: the food you eat shapes the constitution and effectiveness of all your body's mechanisms. Over the long term, choosing the right foods not only helps prevent illness and disease but also enhances your body's capacity to produce energy and positive moods.

On a more specific, short-term basis, exciting new studies show that certain foods have an immediate impact on your mental state and performance. In experiments conducted by Judith Wurtman, Ph.D., of the Massachusetts Institute of Technology, different groups of subjects ate meals consisting of either protein or carbohydrates, and then were questioned about their mood and tested on their problem-solving abilities. The results of the experiments: those who ate protein reported being more alert and energetic, and they performed significantly better on the tests.

Protein, it turns out, triggers certain neurochemicals in your brain (specifically, dopamine and norepinephrine) that heighten mental alertness and efficiency. By eating a high-protein lunch, in other words, you can fight off afternoon fatigue and maintain top levels of mental acuity throughout the day. That's just one suggestion: many other scientific studies in nutrition offer helpful, intelligent advice for improving your health, energy, and performance.

STEP 3: WORKING OUT TO WORK BETTER

Another activity that can furnish amazing gains in energy, confidence, emotional control, and mental clarity is exercise. In the short term, jumping on a stair-climbing machine or going for a run affords you a burst of energy and positive emotion. Even if you're exhausted from several hours of intense work at your desk, 20 to 30 minutes of aerobic exercise produce changes in your body and brain that totally revitalize you.

In the long term, exercise conditions your body to become a more efficient producer of energy (principally by burning more fat as a fuel source), and to respond more effectively in the face of pressure. Remarkably, regular exercise shapes up your emotional response to adversity in the same way it shapes up your ability to run a 3-mile race. Just as a few months of training enables you to breathe easier and run more comfortably, it allows you to greet challenges at work with greater confidence and composure.

Additionally, working out boosts your mental performance. "The brain is a physical organ, and its fitness is dependent upon the fitness of the body in which it resides," says neurologist Michael J. Kushner. Aerobic exercise, as a number of studies have shown, helps you think better, remember more, and react more quickly. Overall, it's an indispensable ally in the campaign to maintain top performance.

STEP 4: BREAKING UP STRESS AND FATIGUE

The fourth step for maintaining your peak mental state is to re-orchestrate your daily schedule, planning in breaks to relax your mind and refresh your energy. Each person's energy cycle—like his or her reaction to food—is unique. But in general (as Dr. Ernest Rossi, author of *The 20-Minute Break*, and many other re-searchers have demonstrated), the body and brain work accord-ing to a process of energy expenditure and then recovery, and aligning your work schedule with this process allows you to oper-ate at your most alert and effective.

In terms of your day at work, most people experience a natural downturn in the midmorning and midafternoon. And unfortu-nately, most people force themselves to work right through these low-energy periods. While that kind of drive is impressive, it ulti-mately defeats the purpose by driving down your productivity and alertness. Especially with the heightened tension and com-plex problems of today's world of work, you're much better off tak-ing a strategic break that allows you to come back with recharged vitality, renewed perspective, and increased productivity.

By understanding the stress and recovery principle—the man-ner in which your body and mind function optimally through pe-riods of exerting energy interspersed with periods of rest and recovery of energy—you can figure out how best to organize your work, rest, meals, and sleep to maintain an optimal energy level and mood.

STEP 5: LEARNING TO LOVE PROBLEMS

Step 5 involves adopting the challenge response to problems, transforming tension into determination and enthusiasm. Even in the face of obstinate problems, headaches, and hardship, you can control your emotions, your energy levels, and your ability to find humor in the world around you. When it comes down to it, you ultimately have the ability to choose your mentality, and how you perceive and react to each situation you encounter. As humor expert Dr. Harvey Mindess postulates, "Our lives, I propose, extend between the poles of tragedy and comedy, but we possess more freedom than we realize to experience our circumstances and ourselves in comic or tragic guise."

The trouble is that—especially in the face of adversity—we "forget to remember" (as the poet e. e. cummings put it) that we possess this freedom. People tend to respond to a reorganization or a new competitor by growing tense, frustrated, or angry. Or maybe even more commonly, by what I call *tanking*—withdrawing all emotional investment from work, going through the motions of your job with no real interest or passion. In today's environment, when problem solving requires knowledge, energy, and ideas, these negative emotions dash your chances of succeeding by choking off the mental dexterity and enthusiasm required to create great products and services. Too tired, too frustrated, or too serious, many people fail to see the possibilities of their situation and allow external events to dictate how they feel and behave.

The key to solving problems is to become not upset, but challenged by the situation. Rather than reacting with frustration, anger, blame, or self-pity, you have to adopt an enthusiastic mindset, see yourself as an expert problem solver, and use the challenge to propel yourself forward to new breakthroughs. Like Sherlock Holmes, you have to engage problems with excitement, tenacity, and a healthy sense of enjoyment.

STEP 6: PUTTING HUMOR TO WORK

Another tactic to infuse dedication, demolish stress, and put yourself in a peak emotional state is to enliven your sense of humor. Vastly underrated as a means of tolerating the ambiguity of business and remaining poised in the face of impossible situations, having a sense of humor—undertaking your tasks in a spirit of joy and challenge—plays an indispensable role in working at your best. "There's no reason that work has to be suffused with seriousness," says Southwest Airlines' immensely successful CEO Herb Kelleher. "Professionalism can be worn lightly. Fun is a stimulant to people. They enjoy their work more and work more productively."

Having fun at work is not just *acceptable.* In today's high-stress atmosphere, fun is an absolute must. Bringing humor into your work enhances enjoyment, dissipates tension, and engenders a heightened state of perspective and control. Biochemically, this happens when laughter sends pleasure-enhancing neurochemicals leaping joyfully through your system. Emotionally, having fun re-awakens passion, stirs excitement, and drives the vigor of your thinking and ideas.

How do you "get funny"? It's not as straightforward as changing your diet. But by surrounding yourself with humorous material—filling your office with jokes, cartoons, comedy videos, funny newsletters and e-mail, amusing pictures and objects—and by actively cultivating your ability to perceive the humor in situations, you can put yourself in the state of mind that drives top performance.

STEP 7: CREATING ENERGIZING ENVIRONMENTS

The final step for engendering an optimal mind-set involves the orchestration of your physical workplace. The typical office—at home or in corporate headquarters—is drab, humorless, and devoid of inspiration. And when your job involves taking bold risks, inventing spine-tingling products, and innovating electrifying new ways to gain market share, that kind of environment just doesn't cut it.

To foster healthy, positive habits of mind and body, you have to modify your physical workplace. As briefly mentioned, humorizing the office can go a long way toward upping the interest and excitement levels. Reminders of past victories and sterling achievements, in addition, can reinforce confidence. Further, you can make many other changes to the office arrangement, furniture, decor, pictures, music, and bulletin boards to boost energy and positive emotions, converting your workplace into a nest of stimulation.

Seize the Day

In today's world of work, you have to confront a vast array of new pressures and challenges. But even while stressful and demanding, this is a time of expanding horizons and limitless opportunities. Realizing the promise of the new world, however, calls for a new approach—new habits, new plans, and new attitudes. As Abraham Lincoln declared when facing a comparable moment of change and urgency, "The dogmas of the quiet past are inadequate to the stormy present. The occasion is piled high with difficulty, and we must rise with the occasion. As our case is new, so we must think anew, and act anew."

Adopting new habits that foster energy and confidence helps prepare you to embrace whatever challenges this new world offers by enabling you to operate at your most imaginative and effective. But more than simply giving you the means to work longer and more efficiently, the CatchFire program helps you unleash the energy, enthusiasm, and enterprise that allow you to gain a measure of satisfaction and enjoyment from your work and life. By reinvigorating your body and mind, you not only tackle your work with greater energy and creativity, you also—as the mythologist Joseph Campbell put it—more fully engage yourself in the "experience of being alive."

> *"Let a man in a garret but burn with enough intensity and he will set fire to the world."*
>
> Antoine de Saint-Éxupéry

"He barks for the love of barking."

THE CATCHFIRE MODEL
Setting the Mind on Fire: The Energy Zone

The greatest discovery of my generation is that human beings can alter their lives by altering their attitudes of mind. —William James

"When you do something," the famous Zen master Shun-ryu Suzuki says, "if you fix your mind on the activity with some confidence, the quality of your state of mind is the activity itself. When you are concentrated on the quality of your being, you are prepared for the activity."

While "quality" programs have spread through thousands of companies in the last decade, the typical corporate climate of pressure and change undermines one of the central components of such initiatives: *the mind-set of the people who make the business work.* Of course, skillfully wrought systems provide a blueprint for success and allow people to channel their energy where it will produce the greatest results. But in addition to an attractive organizational chart, there has to be a certain emotion, mentality, or fire in people that drives excellence and innovation. Inventing breakthrough products, concocting masterful project plans, creating solid client relationships—these acts are born, forged, and consummated from the energy and ingenuity of human beings. They depend, ultimately, on the spark of a focused, energized mind.

Many of the most capable executives in the country view setting the organizational tone—creating a mood characterized by energy, a self-confident mind-set, and a positive sense of urgency—as their single most important role. A notable example is Bernie Marcus, the cofounder and CEO of The Home Depot, who has guided his company with such success that its stock price has skyrocketed 28,000 percent since its inception. "This is not a numbers company. It's an emotional company—emotion drives Home Depot," Marcus said in *Fortune* magazine. "Keeping the spirit alive is the most difficult task we have." At Microsoft, the mentality factor emerges as the dominant consideration for prospective employees. While interested in the knowledge base of a new recruit, Microsoft bases its decisions on whether the candidate possesses energy, enthusiasm, and a prejudice toward creatively attacking problems. For Herb Kelleher, CEO of Southwest Airlines, attitude—with an emphasis on a lively sense of fun—is the main criterion for hiring people. "What we look for, first and foremost, is a sense of humor. Then we are looking for people who have to excel to satisfy themselves," says Kelleher. "We hire attitudes."

The Power of a Positive Mind-set

While you obviously need the appropriate knowledge and skills to do your job, the mind-set with which you approach your work plays a dominant role in your ability to perform. If you're discouraged, you work sluggishly, think small, and give up easily. When you're stressed out, you communicate poorly and can't focus; you may work at a feverish pitch, but you create as many problems as you solve. If you're low on energy, you shun problems, contribute few ideas, and lethargically carry out your assignments. On the other hand, when you're feeling confident, focused, and exhilarated, the world is in your hands. You assemble brilliant ideas, win people to your side, and pull off dazzling projects. Even when intimidating obstacles arise, you greet them with determination and humor, and use them as fodder for break-throughs and triumphs.

When I mention attitudes or states of mind, I'm not talking about something in the metaphysical realm. Your mental and emotional state has biological roots. Getting anxious pitches your body into a state characterized by tense muscles, rapid breathing, elevated heart rate, and high levels of the chemicals epinephrine and norepinephrine—changes that disrupt your ability to think clearly and work effectively. In terms of your brain circuitry, cer-tain emotions cause your brain to selectively remember events in the past associated with those emotions. Thus, feeling depressed calls up earlier failures and misfortunes (a terrible interview, a bad relationship, or an embarrassing presentation in your college speech class). Feeling confident, on the other hand, brings to mind past victories and outstanding performances (your biggest business deal, best presentation, or the brilliant performance at your high school soccer championship game).

Further, when you're in a certain state of mind—whether opti-mistic or discouraged—your brain expects to stay that way. It tunes in to the aspects of the current situation that reinforce its emotional disposition. If you're feeling great, for example, you tend to overlook the troubles and potential disasters inherent in your project, and instead focus on the ways that it can succeed. It's not that you disregard the negative possibilities, but you look past them in a positive way, the way a basketball team ignores the fact that they're down by 20 points and goes on to win the game, or the way Lee Iacocca brushed aside the fact that Chrysler was bankrupt and turned the company around to become a thriv-ing success. Your state of mind isn't inconsequential; it actively shapes the biochemistry of your system and the neural circuitry of your brain.

And this physiological reshaping powerfully influences your ability to perform at work. Positive states of mind—those charac-terized by confidence, enthusiasm, and a healthy sense of hu-mor—boost your brainpower. As Daniel Goleman, Ph.D., says in

Emotional Intelligence, "Good moods enhance the ability to think flexibly and with more complexity, thus making it easier to find solutions to problems, whether intellectual or interpersonal." A positively energized state of mind drives your best planning and decision making.

Cultivating Your Consciousness

Despite the awesome influence of your mind-set, few people effectively control their internal state. While knowing what a vast difference exists between times when they are confident and enthusiastic and times when they are frustrated and lethargic, only a small number of people have learned to put themselves into a positive, productive state of mind when facing difficult situations. The opposite is more nearly the case: most people—even highly intelligent people—regularly work themselves into states that undermine their ability to work effectively.

To perform at your highest level, to maximize the productivity and creativity of the time you spend at work (and to fully enjoy the experience of life), you have to—as the Zen master Shunryu Suzuki says—concentrate on the quality of your state of mind. With the continual changes in business, frustration is easy. Getting stressed out almost comes naturally. But maintaining your optimism and lively sense of humor takes work. You have to make a disciplined effort to put yourself in a positive mind-set, approach your problems with poise and enthusiasm, and continuously renew your sense of humor and passion. You're not just more pleasant in such a state; you change your physiology in a way that improves your ability to create success.

The Professional Workforce Survey put the idea in concrete numbers: people who adopt a positive mind-set toward their job reported themselves to be far more effective than their negative-minded counterparts. Most people, it turned out, reported that they have at least a moderately positive mentality—36 percent "strongly agreed" and another 40 percent "somewhat agreed" they had a positive attitude about their jobs. Comparing the group with a positive attitude to the group without a positive attitude revealed dramatic differences. Those with a positive mentality were almost three times as likely to report high levels of energy. By a measure of 58 percent to 12 percent, more of those with a positive temperament felt a sense of control in their jobs. Further, the positive group was less than half as likely to report feeling high levels of stress and twice as likely to say they could easily pull themselves out of a bad mood (40 percent of the negatively minded said they could lift themselves out of the doldrums, compared to 80 percent of the more upbeat professionals). Maybe most interesting, compared to just over one-fifth of those sporting a bad attitude, almost one-half of the positive-minded strongly agreed that they were top performers at work.

What State Are You In?

In *The Myth of Sisyphus*, the French author Albert Camus suggests that the first thing you should do every morning is to ask yourself whether or not you should commit suicide. (If you can get past that one, then have a great day.) Camus's intention is to get in your face. He forces you to ask yourself if you are committing a sort of philosophical suicide—going through the motions of life without any passion or zest. If you're not pushing as much humor, joy, and fun as possible into each day of your life, then why go through it?

In a similar way, I want you to consider your attitude and behavior at work. What state are you in when you walk into the office? Do you bound into the office ready to make extraordinary things happen? When you answer the phone, are you prepared to have a quick-witted, engaging, or perhaps hilarious conversation? To help you get a clearer idea of what mind-set you take to work, take a look at the following chart. While there are an infinite number of moods or mental states, the four *performance zones* listed here represent some of the most common states people fall into on the job. The schema is simple, but so is the point: to force you to confront your normal mind-set and the effect it has on your job and life.

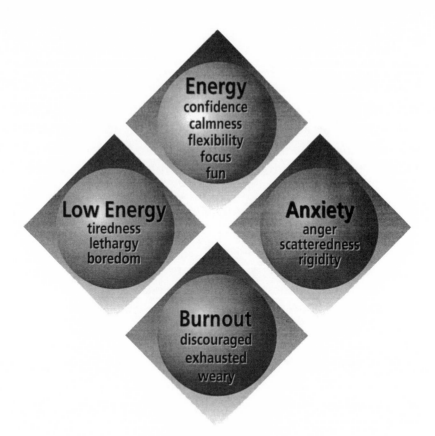

PERFORMANCE ZONES

The *energy zone* is the goal, the attitude that mentally, emotionally, and physiologically helps you perform at your best. Of course, there is no single mentality or personality that guarantees success. I've worked with a variety of successful salespeople, entrepreneurs, and leaders who exhibit starkly different attitudes toward their jobs and lives. But combining knowledge of the demands of today's world of work with scientific evidence of how the body and brain function optimally gives a great deal of insight into what emotions and attitudes lead to outstanding performance. The energy zone describes the state in which you have maximum physical vitality, peak levels of mental alertness and clarity, and an optimal degree of emotional confidence, resilience, and joy. Cultivating this mind-set enables you to consistently meet your circumstances—daunting though they may be—with all of your talent and ingenuity.

This doesn't mean that you have to receive divine inspiration before tackling your phone calls or achieve total enlightenment before you get down to work. In fact, the courage to dive in and make something happen—even if it's a leap in the dark—is a cardinal virtue. But by understanding how your quality of mind influences your thinking and your actions, and by learning the CatchFire strategies to manage your energy and emotions, you can dramatically improve your ability to perform on the job and prosper in life.

The Energy Zone

The energy zone (shown below) is a model, a practical outline of the mentality you need to meet the personal demands of a complex, changing world of business. While other qualities remain important, these qualities represent the most necessary attributes of outstanding performance:

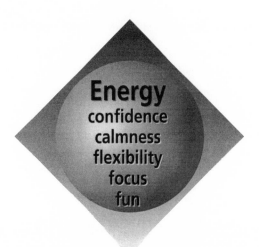

Learning this "script" for a positive mind-set—attuning your internal state to it as an actor internalizes his lines—enables you to retain your composure and your ability to act effectively, no matter what the external circumstances. Possessed of these characteristics, you operate in your optimal state of mind and perform in the upper limits of your ability.

ENERGY

If I were a heathen, I would rear a statue to energy, and fall down and worship it. —Mark Twain

Jack Welch, CEO of General Electric, and the late Roberto Goizueta, former CEO of Coca-Cola, will doubtlessly be remembered as two of the most effective business leaders of our time. Under their supervision, GE and Coca-Cola have each successfully revamped their organizational structures, vastly expanded their global operations, and realized remarkable gains in innovation and productivity. In terms of the creation of shareholder wealth—one of the most fundamental measures of business performance—the two far outdistance any competitors. As *Fortune* magazine reported in December of 1995, Welch and Goizueta had created a combined $111 billion for their shareholders. (Microsoft, Merck, and Wal-Mart, the closest competitors, lagged some distance behind.)

Although these exceptional leaders achieved their success in very different businesses, they agreed completely on the single most important personal quality to thriving in a tumultuous world.

WELCH: "Somebody with incredible energy."

GOIZUETA: "Energy is number one."

In various cultures and historical periods, energy has been characterized as the ultimate mover of things, the prime force of the universe, the fundamental source of action. Such concepts as spirit, prana, chi, *n/um* (the idea of psychophysical energy of the !Kung bushmen of the Kalahari Desert), and life force all describe a power very similar to what we call energy. Physicists, though generally in awe of its properties and forms, have a less transcendental definition of it: the capacity to do work. All senses of the word, however, capture the central idea of the aliveness, strength, and vitality of body and mind that enable you to live fully and initiate vigorous action toward whatever endeavor you choose to pursue.

Energy is the key to motivating yourself, to inculcating excitement into your work and into the people around you, and to enthusiastically persevering in your efforts despite setbacks and problems. It is the wellspring of bold ideas and the fuel that sustains the steadfast pursuit of converting those ideas into reality.

Without question, you need knowledge, experience, and skills to make your energy productive. But as Tim Romani says, raw energy is often the preeminent factor. Serving as Project Executive for the new Pepsi Center in Denver—an arena that will be home to the Denver Nuggets and Colorado Avalanche—Romani faces a monumental, multiplex operation. As he says, "You have to have a certain level of education and experience, but I think more importantly, these projects require an enormous amount of energy." In other words, many times the complex demands of your work reduce to this: can you summon the energy to plow through your arduous project, to make five more calls to prospective clients, to do what it takes to push your proposal through to fruition? The relationship of energy and performance is basic and undeniable: more energy allows you to accomplish more and to attend to your tasks with greater imagination and care. "You can't get tired, because if you do you can miss a lot and make some critical mistakes," says Romani. "The key to any project is to stay on top of it, don't be afraid to make decisions, and have fun because you want to have positive energy and be able to enjoy the ride."

Energy stems from a number of different sources, both psychological and physiological. Every step in the CatchFire program addresses the problem directly or indirectly, including methods to cultivate the attitudes and humor that inspire energetic performance; advice on how you can eat, exercise, and sleep for optimal physical vitality; and ways to create an environment that generates a heightened sense of excitement.

CONFIDENCE

Confidence is that feeling by which the mind embarks in great and honorable courses with a sure hope and trust in itself. —Cicero

The word *confidence* comes from the Latin *con* and *fidens*, which literally mean "with faith." Having faith in yourself doesn't mean that your circumstances never unsettle you or cause you to doubt your judgments. It indicates instead a general self-assuredness, an inner belief that you will be able to successfully solve the problems—even if formidable—that confront you.

The most important element of confidence is a sense of optimism. Optimism refers to a mentality defined by hope and the simple expectation that you will accomplish what you set out to do. While no one works completely free from periods of self-doubt or worry, a sense of optimism helps in eradicating this kind of performance-crippling thinking, replacing it with such a strong orientation toward success that problems seem to willingly yield their solutions. Particularly important when working in a position where the rate of failure is high, optimism enables you to persist through difficult times, unfazed by setbacks and defeats.

More than a mere sensation, this orientation plays a major role in the quality of your thinking and performance. As Albert Bandura, a Stanford psychologist and leading researcher on self-efficacy, says, "People's beliefs about their abilities have a profound effect on those abilities. Ability is not a fixed property; there is a huge variability in how you perform. People who have a sense of self-efficacy bounce back from failures; they approach things in terms of how to handle them rather than worrying about what can go wrong."

A second aspect of confidence involves staying composed when the heat is on, retaining your mental agility and toughness under pressure. Critical when deliberating in an intense negotiation, giving a pivotal presentation to a crowd of exacting executives, or wending your way through the closing session of a major sale, the ability to stay composed can make the difference between success and failure.

Confidence comes, in large part, from competence, practice, and preparation. But it also results from your habits of thinking and your physical and physiological states. I mentioned the potent force of optimism in maintaining a confident mentality, but the way you interpret your successes and failures also plays a critical role in your ability to stay confident. (Not accepting the usual negative explanations we give ourselves when a project goes bad, research says, is a vital—and learnable—characteristic of confident people.) Another interesting component of confidence is your physical posture. When your back is straight, your shoulders back, and your muscles relaxed, your body sends physiological messages to your brain that create a confident attitude. Lastly, along with an optimistic disposition and an assertive physical bearing, physical exercise plays a vital role in creating the biochemistry of confidence. Learning to control these dispositions of mind and body greatly enhances your confidence, and hence your ability to perform.

CALMNESS

If your mind is calm and constant, you can keep yourself away from the noisy world even though you are in the midst of it. In the midst of noise and change, your mind will be quiet and stable. —Shunryu Suzuki

In *Zen and the Art of Motorcycle Maintenance*, Robert Pirsig extols the wisdom of a Japanese bicycle assembly manual that begins, "Assembly of Japanese bicycle require great peace of mind." Knowing that most people struggle mightily with such a project, the instruction manual aims to overcome the number one barrier to successful assembly: the frustration and turmoil of the assembler's mind. "The ultimate test's always your own serenity," Pirsig says. "If you don't have this when you start and maintain it while you're working you're likely to build your personal problems right into the machine itself."

Serenity seems in preciously short supply today, a casualty of the unrelenting assault of information, technology, and competition. To keep up, many organizations emphatically advocate its opposite, urging a "disdain for complacency," a "healthy paranoia," or a "sense of urgency." Instilling this kind of bias toward action helps create a productive corporate culture. But often it promotes a serious negative consequence: it extinguishes a sense of calmness, a relaxed self-possession that is vital for optimal thinking and decision making.

While seemingly inconsistent with excitement and activity, a sense of calmness engenders a cool, lucid mind that enables you to work efficiently under stress. Perhaps most important when dealing with crisis situations, an inner calmness affords you the critical ability to make good decisions in a fast-paced, frantic, and imperfect world. Rather than getting tense under pressure, and building that tension into your team or your work, you perform a sort of mental judo and calmly defuse the stress. (*Judo* literally means "the art of soft falling," a discipline in which you use the energy of your opponent to politely whirl him over on his back.) With greater emotional stability and enhanced clarity of mind— when energized and calm rather than energized and frenetic— you communicate more effectively, think more expansively, and work far more productively.

As Dr. Herbert Benson points out in *The Relaxation Response*, almost every culture in history had some mechanism (such as prayer, meditation, or yoga) or some regular period in the day devoted to relaxation—a time in which people rested their bodies and quieted their minds. Unfortunately, Benson says, "our society has given very little attention to the importance of relaxation." The result? Physiologically, we generate excessive levels of the "stress" hormones epinephrine and cortisol, and our health suffers from escalated rates of hypertension and heart disease. Psychologically, many of us go through life high-strung and agitated, with the chronic feeling that we'll never catch up. Not only is this condition unpleasant, it hinders your body's ability to generate energy and severely impairs your ability to perform.

Developing inner calmness requires, first and foremost, reincorporating periods of relaxation into your day. In upcoming chapters, we discuss the most beneficial times in the day for such "recovery periods," as well as the most effective physical and mental exercises—including breathing exercises, relaxation techniques, stretching, and aerobic exercise—to promote a loose and balanced frame of mind.

FLEXIBILITY

To be a man of knowledge one must be fluid and light.   —Yaqui mystic

Flexibility of thinking and action has characterized many ground-breaking leaders and innovators. But until recently, the ability to be flexible mattered little in most occupations. A few decades ago, not only did the average "organizational man" work his whole life for the same company, he worked with the same group of people, providing the same products and services for the same customers. Soon after you began working for one corporation or another, you could confidently map out your career path in its entirety, charting your rise to, say, production floor supervisor or regional vice president at age 45 or 50—a position in which you could coast until retirement. The permanence and pre-dictability of that world stand in astonishing contrast to the situation today.

Change is the dominant feature of today's landscape. And continual change means that, in addition to being energetic and poised, you have to be flexible. More than merely an admirable trait, the ability to flexibly adapt and dive into new situations has become an essential element to great performance—and even to survival.

Flexibility entails a nimble mind and an emotional disposition of resilience and openness. It suggests the willingness to un-freeze your fixed set of expectations and forsake any tendency to cling to rigid structures. Emotionally, flexible people display a highly developed tolerance for ambiguity and the ability to absorb the confusion and frustration of a fast-paced environ-ment without becoming tight and tense. Mentally, flexibility in-volves the capacity to carry your assumptions lightly, to rise above intellectual tunnel vision, and to entertain a more expansive array of options. Finally, being flexible allows you to respond creatively in the face of stressful change, to react adroitly to unavoidable

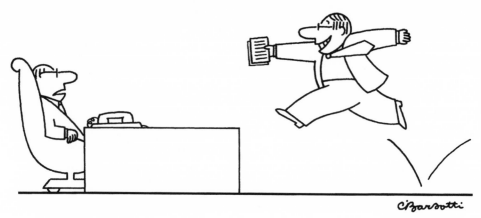

"You had damn well better not be putting a good face on bad news, Wilson."

problems and new roles—in fact, to see the new opportunities presented by them.

Glenda Haines, a manager in the marketing department of Public Service Company of Colorado, knows intimately the shock of major change ("Our business is really going through a complete revolution—I don't think it's transitional change") and the consequent need to remain flexible. Public Service, like utility companies across the nation, is grappling with the deregulation of the industry, a development that portends the end of its natural monopoly and the beginning of becoming a truly market driven organization. Predictably, deregulation has initiated a trend of downsizings and mergers, one of which involves the future combination of Public Service of Colorado with Southwest Public Service of Texas. "I'm always telling my department that we've got to remain flexible. We don't know what kind of thinking is going to come from the merger teams, and how they think things should go together. But if the work we're doing is valuable, that's what we've got to count on—not a position, not an organizational structure."

For Haines, it's not just a speech for her employees. Along with almost everybody in the corporation, she had to reapply for a job after being erased from the organizational chart two years ago, a procedure she describes as "complicated, fearful, and emotionally stressful." Looking to the upcoming merger, she says she will undoubtedly need to retain her ability to flexibly adapt: "I feel like I'm in the most vulnerable position, because I don't believe my job will exist after the merger. But I believe that there will be great job opportunities, and I feel very good about my opportunity to have one of those."

FOCUS

Concentration is the secret of strength in politics, in war, in trade, in short, in all management of human affairs. —Ralph Waldo Emerson

Focus defines the ability to concentrate your thinking and action toward one specific object, to hone in on something with optimal alertness. Always a critical quality for success, burgeoning workloads and an inundation of information have made the capacity to focus a matter of life or death. A good metaphor for this characteristic is the way a magnifying glass focuses sunlight on a piece of paper: the lens takes the dispersed energy of sun rays and zeroes them in on a single point—a solitary nucleus of intensity—that quickly produces a flicker of flame, a trail of smoke, and a burned-out hole.

There are two different but interrelated elements that constitute a successfully focused mind. The first involves something like the mental concentration of an athlete. In addition to alertness, clarity, and calmness of mind, focus means the ability to silence external distractions, quiet internal mental chatter, and immerse yourself in the implications and possibilities of an issue. It requires that you rid your consciousness of the thousand things you have to do and concentrate your mind right here, right now, on the project at hand. Like a cat ready to pounce on a bird, like a basketball player at the free throw line, a focused mind singles out its task from the vast universe and calmly, purposefully intends its every effort toward that task's accomplishment.

The second aspect of focus concerns a longer-term direction of your energy and thinking—focusing on specific projects to achieve specific meaningful goals. The temptation to do urgent things constantly eats at everyone. Working effectively, however, requires focus.

Steve Baldwin, a senior partner at Deloitte & Touche Consulting Group, says that focus is critical in a business environment that resembles a scramble. "It's the analogy of the *Ed Sullivan Show* and the guy with all the sticks spinning plates on top, running back and forth to keep them all spinning," says Baldwin. "We all have to deal with that." As his team assists a Fortune 100 company in a total overhaul of their corporate structure—one of the biggest projects Deloitte & Touche Consulting Group has ever undertaken—Baldwin says that the ability to focus is invaluable: "Even though life is complex and there are many aspects to the project, you have to be able to zero in on one bit, drill down and engage, and put it to bed. You have to focus on something and drive it to completion in a fairly short time frame, get it done and out of the way."

Focus is intricately connected with two things. First, focus requires balanced blood sugar levels, maintained primarily by eating the right foods at the right times. And second, focus follows fun—when you're joyfully engaged in a project, your attentive powers are concentrated at their peak.

FUN

We're all working harder and faster. But unless we're also having more fun, the transformation doesn't work.   —Jack Welch, CEO, General Electric

In studies of peak performances, nearly all the various "performers" reported that they intensely enjoyed the experience, whether it was a violin concerto, ski jump, business deal, or chess match. Some tough-minded people labor under the illusion that work is a process of gritty, grueling, painful struggle. These people have a point, of course: sometimes you have to force yourself to accomplish arduous tasks or deal with highly unpleasant people. But in an economy where value derives from networks, knowledge, and ideas, the race goes to the passionate and witty rather than the grim and plodding. Undertaking your work with a sense of play fuels enthusiasm, builds relationships, and sparks the ability to become challenged and engaged in response to problems, instead of angry or threatened.

Fun (if you haven't had any in a while) describes a general feeling of enjoyment, an enthusiastic involvement in the task at hand. While sometimes it includes passionate feelings of zest, one indispensable element of fun is a sense of playfulness. I don't mean playful as in possessed of a silly, frolicsome personality, but playful as in having a sense of lightheartedness and a keen awareness of the bountiful possibilities inherent in every situation (even those disguised as insoluble problems). Seemingly a matter of less than vital importance, the capacity to perceive humor and joy in your job turns out to serve many crucial purposes. In a world dominated by overly serious people doing sterile work, the state of fun liquidates anxiety while spurring vitality and creativity. It engenders the sporting, adventuresome attitude that allows you to treat problems as games, to view crises as contests, and to see breakdowns as breakthroughs.

How can you develop this sense of fun? Humor and laughter—the munitions of mirth—open the door to a state of joy and zest. Incorporating jokes, cartoons, and various other sources of humor into your meetings, your office, and your life continually reminds you of the gamelike quality of existence. Biochemically, laughter triggers a response similar to exercise, sending messenger molecules coursing happily through your system to create a healthy, animated state of body and mind. But while thunderous belly laughs give your physiology a vigorous shake, you don't have to traipse about pretending you're Bill Cosby; the most important goal is to cultivate your appreciation of the comic side of business and life. As the historian Conrad Hyers says, "Getting the point of a joke is not the same as getting the point of joking."

In the Zone

To crystallize the concept of the energy zone, compare your ability to perform at times when you don't have these six attributes of mind to your ability to perform when they're all present. When you're tired and sluggish, for example—when you lack energy, focus, and a sense of fun—your effectiveness diminishes in every aspect of your work. Your productivity plummets, your ability to communicate dwindles, and your ideas emerge grudgingly and lifeless. If a problem surfaces, you will very likely engage in a series of acts such as complaining, blaming, ignoring, and denying (we hope you've given up kicking and cursing) before you get around to trying to solve it. A comparable breakdown occurs if you're overwhelmed by stress: you lose your ability to concentrate, you tend to think rigidly, and your sense of composure decays to a state of frantic hyperactivity or helpless inaction.

On the other end of the spectrum—when you're in the energy zone—you feel pumped, psyched, jazzed, and otherwise unstoppable. Working with confidence and focus, radiating enthusiasm and joy—in this mode, you make the seemingly impossible look easy. You spur forward projects, you conceive breakthrough concepts, you engineer victories and take pleasure in doing it. The psychologist Abraham Maslow, in his book *Towards a Psychology of Being*, used the term *fully-functioning* to describe how people perform when they have this attitude. "What takes effort, straining and struggling at other times," Maslow writes, "is now done without any sense of striving, of working or laboring, but 'comes of itself.' Allied to this often is the feeling of effortless fully-functioning, when everything 'clicks,' or 'is in the groove,' or is 'in overdrive.' "

The Physiology of Emotion

The energy zone depicts what people usually consider to be a state of mind, a combination of your thinking patterns and your emotions. Most people consider a "state of mind" to be ephemeral—a condition that can come or go, a mood that can overtake or desert you. Advances in mind/body science, however, demonstrate that emotions or states of mind have specific, measurable reflections in biochemistry. In other words, a certain state of mind corresponds to a certain biochemical state, and further, a change in one induces a change in the other. So by improving

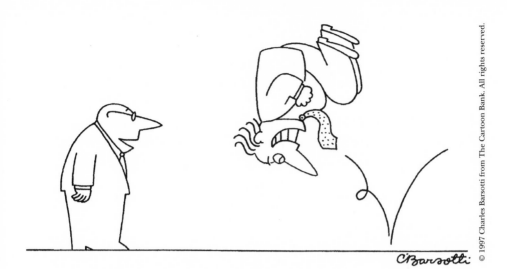

"See, there, Perkins, I told you if you switched from three-martini lunches to a high-carbohydrate diet you'd feel perkier in the afternoons."

your mind-set, you can alter your biochemistry to a more healthy, positive state. And on the other side of the coin, by altering your biochemistry (by such activities as exercising, deep breathing, eating, relaxing, laughing, and sleeping), you can effectively alter your state of mind.

While there isn't a precisely known biochemical state that leads to peak levels of thinking and action, possessing the attributes described by the energy zone creates the biochemistry that fosters sharp thinking, emotional control, and the ability to work effectively. More specifically, having a positive mind-set modifies the "stress response" with which evolution has endowed you. Instead of stimulating the biochemical changes that lead to nervousness or anger (the anxiety zone), being in the energy zone enables you to react to your demands with an appropriate response, whether that means a calm demeanor or a fighting spirit.

Stressed Out or Fired Up?

When confronted by a challenging situation—an impending deadline, an angry client, a dissatisfying relationship, or any event that requires a mental, physical, or emotional response—your mind and body automatically go through a number of physiological changes that prepare themselves to handle it. The adrenal glands secrete the stress hormones epinephrine (also called adrenaline) and norepinephrine, which induce an increased heart rate, higher blood glucose levels, an accelerated metabolic rate, and other reactions that provide you with more available energy and improved abilities to think clearly and act quickly. This is an ingrained response with which evolution has equipped us, a response that allowed our ancestors to fight or flee when faced with threatening situations (in the form of a hungry dinosaur or an erupting volcano). Beyond this generic response, there are two modified but still general reactions produced by your body and mind. The first is to become negatively aroused or "stressed out"; the second involves responding with positive energy, optimistic thinking, and a fighting spirit—a "fired up" response that embodies the feelings and attitudes described by the energy zone.

The experience of feeling stressed out—anxious, strained, frustrated, and fearful—affects almost everyone in this hurried environment of business (as noted previously, 70 percent of the working population agreed that stress negatively affects their health and performance). When in this state of negative arousal, the ingrained physiological response of your system works against you, producing a biochemical response suitable for fending off a woolly mammoth, but totally inappropriate for tactfully turning around a disinterested buyer. The adrenal glands secrete excessive levels of epinephrine and norepinephrine, as well as a hormone called cortisol, which results in scattered thinking, erratic decisions, and ineffective if not counterproductive interaction with other people.

The second response—becoming positively aroused in the face of stressful situations—produces a different effect on your biochemistry and an entirely different effect on your performance. In fact, when you face your problems and tasks with the positive mind-set of the energy zone, you allow your body to tailor its biochemical production to the situation at hand. When confronted by emotionally trying circumstances—circumstances in which heightened levels of arousal would do you no good—your biochemical state helps you to handle them with coolness and poise. In the midst of an argument at a meeting, for example, your body secretes a lower amount of epinephrine and norepinephrine, which allows you to remain calm and composed. On the other hand, in the face of a novel situation that requires quick thinking and action, you produce higher than normal levels of epineph-rine and norepinephrine, which enables you to manage the event with more energy and brainpower. In either case, mastering a positive mind-set helps you create a state of biochemistry that allows you to make better decisions and work more productively.

Again, the exciting part of this science lies in the fact that, by adopting habits that induce positive biochemical changes, you can consistently put yourself in the energy zone. And therefore, you can improve your ability to energize a meeting or project, stay calm and confident in the face of menacing deadlines, and maintain towering levels of productivity. Instead of responding to the pressure and change in your job with anxiety or resentment, you can address your problems with optimism and determina-tion, and engage your work with energy, focus, and fun.

Mind Quality Control

The process of gaining control of your mind constitutes one of the most difficult and fundamental challenges you face not only in business, but in life. In order to equip yourself with such con-trol, you have to cultivate new habits of thinking and adopt a healthier, energy-enhancing lifestyle. Many effective tactics to gain control over your energy and mood involve changing your biochemistry through "physical" routines. Thirty minutes of aero-bic exercise, for example, can renew your energy and invigorate your thinking. Eating a high-protein lunch helps you maintain alertness throughout the afternoon. A 5-minute deep-breathing exercise can replace nervousness with a sense of calm and confi-dence. While these habits dramatically improve your ability to thrive in your job, however, they subsume themselves under the paramount strategy: mastering your state of mind and the way you think and feel about the world.

The Power to Choose

It's interesting to remember that for a good part of the history of the Western world, human beings were conceived of as "fixed," with their abilities, mentality, and personality preordained and permanent. Only until relatively recently have we begun to believe that, to a great extent, we have the power to change and improve ourselves. Today, even in the midst of impressive discoveries that demonstrate the significant role of genetics in the way we think and behave, psychological and physiological research supports the notion that, on a fundamental level, you can choose the way you think. That is, you are free to interpret your experiences as hopeless, frustrating, or actually kind of fun, regardless of their "objective" threat or promise. And further, this formulation determines to a great extent your effectiveness at dealing with circumstances—influencing your thinking, decision making, and productivity.

The idea that you can control your mind-set is simple; its practice is far from easy. When you're under severe deadline pressure, taking on the responsibilities of two and a half people, and dealing with a cold, ungrateful boss, most people find it difficult to maintain a sense of composure and enthusiasm. How are you supposed to stay calm with a hectic schedule? What humor could you possibly find in the situation? While exasperation seems the more natural response, remember that nothing is preventing you from seeing your situation as challenging, character building, or comical. As Viktor Frankl wrote in *Man's Search for Meaning*, "We who lived in the concentration camps can remember the men who walked through the huts comforting others, giving away their last piece of bread. They may have been few in number, but they offer sufficient proof that everything can be taken from a man but one thing: The last of his freedoms—to choose one's attitude in any given set of circumstances, to choose one's own way."

Even in the midst of chaos, encountering your problems with confidence, calmness, and flexibility, and seizing your opportunities with energy, focus, and a sense of fun, creates the biochemistry and positive emotions that propel optimal performance.

CATCHFIRE TIPS TO SET YOUR MIND ON FIRE

1. Learn the six elements of the energy zone.
2. Ask yourself, at several intervals over the course of the day: What state am I in?
3. Before a meeting or presentation, ask yourself: Am I energetic, confident, calm, flexible, focused, and fun?
4. Recognize when you're anxious or lethargic, and assume the characteristics of the energy zone.
5. Choose your mentality, no matter what the circumstances.

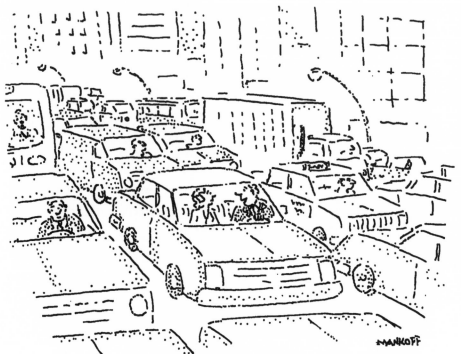

"Hey, is this great traffic, or what?"

STEP 1
Mastering Your Mind: To See with Fresh Eyes

Changes in the technology and organizations of society tend to anesthetize us, to dim our awareness. What we need is a newly awakened perception of what is now going on and a vision of what could.

—Harvey Cox, *The Feast of Fools*

B ill Hewlett and David Packard launched their company in Packard's small, dimly lit garage, with starting capital of $538. Soichiro Honda, whose family was so poor that malnutrition took the lives of five of his siblings, dropped out of the eighth grade to fix old bicycles and pursue his fantasy of building automobiles. Fred Smith and his people at Federal Express lived perilously close to bankruptcy during the early years of the company; Smith himself fought through several blown deals, an indictment for bank fraud, a lawsuit from his family, and his removal from authority (at the hands of his investors) before he finally established the success of the company and his position as its leader.

Looking at the handsome corporate offices, distinctive logos, and impressive year-end reports of Hewlett-Packard, Honda Motors, Federal Express, and other solid, flourishing companies, you get the feeling that they have existed, strongly positioned and well capitalized, since the beginning of time. Unaware of the blind alleys, wrong turns, and dead ends that the leaders of these organizations encountered, you may adopt the notion that they followed a steady, smooth, intelligently planned road to success.

Fumbling Forward

Most roads to success, however, are anything but steady and smooth. At one time, as the classic stories of Hewlett-Packard, Honda, and Federal Express illustrate, all brilliant products and far-flung corporate empires were mere ideas—crazy, foolish ideas in the eyes of many observers—backed by nothing save the hope and perseverance of their originators. Like anyone exploring new territory, these pioneers didn't stroll down a straight road as much as they hacked their way along a labyrinthine path. Progress often consisted in fumbling forward. (On Federal Express's first day of business, for example, the fleet of planes from the East Coast arrived in Memphis to transfer all the packages they had gathered—all *six* of them.) Blunders, crises, and breakdowns occasionally knocked them a few steps back. (Honda's first company, a manufacturer of piston rings, was apparently fated for disaster: a bomb severely damaged the facility in 1945, and an earthquake leveled it a short while later.) Considering the imposing obstacles, make-or-break deals, and near catastrophes faced by these leaders, it's a wonder they ever succeeded.

All this isn't to say their respective journeys weren't fun. Obviously, the likes of Hewlett, Packard, Honda, and Smith had many victories to celebrate. Along with many entrepreneurs, they generally enjoyed hacking their way toward their goals—at times they exhibited an unabashed relish for it. (Amassing a personal fortune of millions, as each managed to do sooner or later, couldn't have hurt.)

Creating Your Own Reality

Forging ideas into reality, whether you are a manager, part of a product design team, or a world leader, often hinges on one over-riding ability: the capacity to consciously maintain a state of hope and belief that propels you forward no matter what the circumstances. The specific problems that need to be resolved may require technological wizardry, engineering expertise, or an aptitude for mobilizing a group of people. The more basic challenge, however, involves a competition with yourself. Can you maintain your expectations of success when the odds are against you? Are you able to stave off feelings of discouragement and defeat, and reassert a sense of optimism and control? Can you recognize when you've been acting with an intolerable degree of serious-ness and desperately need to lighten up? For trailblazing entre-preneurs, as well as any top performer, these issues frequently prove decisive. Winning the internal battle—guiding belief and enthusiasm to victory over doubt and self-reproach—allows you to dive into your challenges with fresh thinking and vigorous ac-tion, even when the situation appears bleak.

There's no easy formula for overcoming doubt and putting yourself into the energy zone. But the first step of the CatchFire program—mastering your mind—will help you drive away dis-couragement and anxiety, and reignite your enthusiasm and determination. As psychological research demonstrates, certain ways of monitoring and directing your thoughts lead to the con-fidence, control, and optimism that inspire top performance. Foremost among these psychological strategies is developing a heightened sense of self-awareness. A major reason people suc-cumb to negative states of mind is that they simply don't pay at-tention to their moods; becoming more attuned to your thoughts and emotions is the key to transforming your mentality to a more productive state. Other key strategies to dispel negative moods and instill optimism involve controlling your self-talk and using visualization. While these practices are indispensable for staying poised in the face of traumatic circumstances—say, your major client switches to your biggest competitor, or an earthquake takes out your office building—they also enhance your ability to think and perform in any situation.

The Professional Workforce Survey demonstrated a clear correlation between managing your thoughts and having a positive mind-set, particularly in the area of managing stress. By a ratio of approximately 2 to 1, people who are well attuned to their attitudes and emotions felt low levels of negative stress compared to those who seldom pay attention to how they're thinking and feeling. Additionally, while only about one-fourth of those who say they are adept at controlling their thoughts and emotions feel high levels of tension, almost two-thirds of those who don't skillfully manage their mind and mood report being very tense. Aside from the enhanced ability to manage their stress levels, most professionals agree that paying attention to their mind-set and directing it to a more positive state helps them work more effectively.

Recognizing the pervasive influence of your thoughts and emotions—and the control you can exercise over them—is an enlightening realization. Essentially, this recognition leads to the fact that by managing your thoughts, you create your own reality. As researchers such as Candace Pert, Ph.D. (the former Chief of Brain Biochemistry of the National Institute of Mental Health), point out, this relationship is reflected on a physiological level. Your perceptions, beliefs, and emotions don't just subtly influence the biochemistry of your brain, they actively create it. In other words, what we pay attention to and allow into our consciousness—whether it's perceptions of anxiety, confident thinking, or feelings of delight—not only affects us psychologically but changes our biology. The power of one's mind-set allows one person to resiliently struggle through her problems—seeing how her situation is not only a good challenge but pretty damn funny, in a way—while another sees nothing but limitations, gets discouraged, and quits. Learning how to wield this power by cultivating your awareness, positive self-talk, and visualization allows you to control your mental state and maximize your performance.

The Age of All-at-Onceness

Managing your state of mind is a vastly more complicated task than it used to be. While today's existence is far less physically precarious than in earlier civilizations, a number of other factors conspire to present a different—but still formidable—challenge to our minds and bodies. In addition to continual changes in business and technology, we live a much faster-paced lifestyle. Daily experience exposes us to unremitting pressure and a dizzying degree of complexity. Tackling prodigious workloads, firing off decisions, and responding to a wealth of letters, e-mails, and voice messages is enough to preoccupy, if not totally overwhelm, the mass of neurons, cells, and electrical circuits that is your brain. Paul Violassi, for example—head of the fast-growing Softech Solutions—makes over 100 phone calls a day to prospective clients. Steve Baldwin, a senior partner at Deloitte & Touche Consulting Group, is bombarded with over 250 e-mails a week. Many people have so much to do, and so much to master, they forfeit any chance for a moment of reflection or introspection.

The result is a feeling of numbness. As though they were perpetually under the strain of finals week, many people seem to have lost their freshness and vivacity. Barry Triller, Executive Vice President at Mutual Life of Canada, says that he regularly encounters people who seem to be overwhelmed. "It's the psychological perception for people that they can never catch up," Triller says. "They're never on top of everything. No matter how much they've done, there's still a pile of work at the end of the day. There are more things to read, and other things they wished they had improved on."

Worse yet, many people don't even realize their predicament. They plow through their days, frantically rescuing this and tending to that, without the recognition that, frankly speaking, they are sapless and flat. "Staleness stalks us" is how Tom Peters puts it in *The Tom Peters Seminar*. He tells a revealing story of his shock, many years ago, at his coworker's decision to take an absurdly long one-month vacation every year. "We were a macho, type-A organization.

I couldn't imagine why he did it. At any rate, I knew that I didn't need a month off, I of boundless energy. Then one year I spent August at a cabin on the Northern California coast. When I got back, I was immediately aware of what a burned-out shell I'd been."

No matter how your business is doing, I imagine the sentiment strikes home. In a hurried and hectic world, it is all too easy to get swept up in the stream of events. Before you realize it, your mind has become its own swift, agitated torrent. Only in sporadic moments of clarity (the kind induced by a month on the beach) do you recognize that you've become tense and edgy, bereft of fresh thinking and a sense of perspective.

Beginner's Mind— Present-Moment Awareness

Breaking the cycle of stress and staleness—the mind-numbing, perspective-narrowing pressure that enfeebles energy and ideas—requires that you develop an enhanced awareness of the present moment. Zen masters refer to this kind of heightened consciousness as *beginner's mind*, meaning a mentality similar to the unassuming, excited, vibrant perspective of a child. When you approach the world with beginner's mind, you shed the dullness and cynicism that have been clouding your view and reawaken your vision of the boundless opportunities for challenge and delight available in every moment. With such a sense of awareness, you can transform a depressingly dull series of phone calls into an interesting game, or a customer complaint into a chance to improve and solidify your relationship with the client.

The process of developing present-moment awareness means learning how to pay closer attention to what is going on right now. That may sound redundant, but I think most people find that, in any given minute, their attention darts like a humming-bird to a hundred different spots—from their relationship with their spouse to their lunch plans to their car problems to the work that is staring them in the face. In fact, a Stanford University study found that a majority of people spend an astounding 58 minutes of every hour thinking about the past or anticipating the future, and only 2 minutes focusing on their present concerns. Again, this is somewhat understandable given today's frantic pace of life. But the nomadic mind is a highly inefficient mind. Learning to focus your mind in the here and now opens you up to enhanced flexibility, greater control, and concentrated thinking. It helps you make better sales calls, work more efficiently, and communicate more effectively with your boss.

Raisin Consciousness

At the Stress Clinic at the University of Massachusetts Medical School, cofounder and director Jon Kabat-Zinn leads an exercise with participants to help them improve present-moment awareness. The exercise does not involve hypnotism, or chanting, or special robes of any kind. The exercise consists in simply this: eating a raisin. But not just popping it in and gulping it down. Rather, eating the raisin in a new way, with total mindfulness and attention, the way a wine connoisseur would sample a vintage Bordeaux. Participants consciously pick the raisin up, observe the color, note its smell, and deliberately place the delicate fruit in their mouth. They feel the folds of its skin on their tongue, its chewiness in between their teeth. They very carefully swallow it, noticing how it feels as it slides down their throat, and savor its distinctive taste. The whole experience, most participants report, is nothing short of dramatic. Immediately, they realize the contrast between approaching an activity with awareness and approaching it in the hasty, unconscious, scatterbrained mode that constitutes the usual manner of existence.

The point of the exercise—the point in becoming more aware of the present moment—is to master your ability to pay attention to the matter at hand. Leaving behind the never-ending worries and distractions about the past, the future, and the course of events over which you have no control—the kind of wasted mental energy that sabotages your vivacity and original thinking—

revitalizes your zest and perspective. Learning to absorb yourself fully in eating a raisin or in formulating a new marketing strategy enables you to devote your peak concentration and most creative thinking to the task at hand.

Posturing for Success— Body Awareness

The yogis and mystics of various Eastern cultures use the body as a tool to help them attain a certain mental state. The lotus position, for example, predisposes the practiced meditator to a relaxed yet alert frame of mind. For the past two or three centuries, Western medicine has largely ignored the fact, but the recent surge in mind/body research is based on the understanding that the brain and body influence each other in extremely significant ways. In fact, more precise terminology wouldn't even make a distinction between the "body" and the "brain." Most people, however, have lost touch with their bodies. They act as if their head rides around on top of their shoulders like a cowboy on top of a stagecoach, oblivious to the fact that what happens to one inextricably affects the other.

Thomas Tierney, cofounder and CEO of Body Wise International, a nutritional supplement company based in southern California, is a devoted believer in the value of becoming more attuned to your body. "If a person will find a quiet space and listen to his or her own body, there are physical feelings in your body you can't ignore that tell you something about what's happening to you," says Tierney. "I know when I receive signals that something isn't quite right, I have to look at not only what events have precipitated it, but if there is a lifestyle change I have to make, like more exercise, fewer business lunches, more walking, or more water drinking."

Becoming more aware of his body actually helped lead Tierney and his partner Ray Grimm to launch Body Wise. As the idea for the company was germinating, Tierney woke up to the fact that he had let his health deteriorate, leaving him overweight, with high cholesterol, and at risk for developing heart disease. Deciding to make a change in his state, Tierney began exercising, eating a very healthy low-fat diet, and taking the nutritional supplements he was creating for their company. Becoming more attuned to his physical and mental well-being and taking the positive steps to change them were critical factors, Tierney says, in allowing him to create the thriving success of his company: after seven years, they have grown into a $60 million organization.

Becoming more aware of how your mind and body interact—for instance, how anxiety causes your breathing to accelerate and your muscles to tense up—is a great way to stay attuned to your state of mind. Sometimes the first imprint on your conscious awareness that you are upset and edgy comes from the realization that your jaw is clenched or you're tapping your foot on the floor like a drummer. Noticing this, you can take a brief moment to relax, reflect on what might be troubling you, and consciously shift yourself from a state of edginess into the energy zone (whether by talking to yourself, visualizing yourself being calm and confident, taking a break, or whipping out a stash of your favorite cartoons). Whether you are in the midst of an important meeting or taking care of routine work at your desk, such a switch shifts you into a higher gear of productivity. Training yourself to notice such signals from your body gives you a great tool to manage your mind.

Becoming aware of your breathing patterns is one of the best methods of body awareness. As you read this, briefly turn your attention to your breathing. Is it on the erratic and shallow side, or is it deep, comfortable, and rhythmic? Whichever it is, you'll find that it corresponds to your mental and emotional state. Irregular, shallow breathing (called *thoracic* breathing because it is concentrated in the thorax in your upper chest) is associated with elevated levels of tension. Deep, comfortable breathing (called *diaphragmatic* because it originates in the diaphragm, near the stomach) accompanies a calm, confident state of mind. As meditators have known for centuries, this practice of focusing on your breath is an amazing way to get a reading on your emotions. And further, the exercise provides you an effective way to take charge of them: take a few deep diaphragmatic breaths through your nose as you read this sentence, and you'll find that you instantly feel more relaxed and more in control. We'll talk more about breathing exercises in Step 4, but for purposes of awareness, remember that a very simple, practical way to enhance your awareness—and make positive changes in your mind-set—is to focus on your breathing and bring it under your control.

Just as breathing is a window to the emotions, your posture tells a great deal about your energy levels and mood. The word *attitude*, in fact, originally described the posture or physical bearing of a sculpture. The disposition of your body literally sends signals to the brain that influence how you think and feel (and vice versa—a certain state of mind sends messages to your body that influence how you carry yourself). Not surprisingly, when in a depressed or fatigued state, you tend to slump down in your chair, your shoulders cave inward, and you tend to focus your eyes downward. To an outside observer, you look discouraged and defeated. Alternatively, sitting upright with your shoulders drawn back is a physical disposition associated with an energetic and confident mind-set. Passersby will at once identify you as a bold visionary, a person of action, and a leader of men.

As with breathing, you can become more cognizant of your attitude by paying closer attention to your posture. Catch yourself, as often as you can, when your shoulders are sagging or your body is bent with tiredness. Straightening yourself up and drawing your shoulders back will transform your mind into a more confident, collected state.

An additional element of becoming more aware of your body is paying more attention to how various foods, exercise, and relaxation periods affect your energy, mood, and performance. Most people pay very little attention to how a third cup of coffee affects their tension level, or how five hours of sleep instead of their usual seven will impact their energy the next day, or how a 10-minute walk influences their ability to think. Too often people go through life tired in the afternoon, and never correlate that with the half-pound burger they eat for lunch. Or they never realize that a midmorning slump in energy might be related to the pastries they munched down for breakfast. Functioning at your peak requires that you experiment, pay attention, and implement the habits that optimize your energy and state of mind.

Standing Behind Yourself— Attitude Awareness

The easiest way to understand the usefulness of a heightened sense of awareness is to recall a situation in which it was absent. Loud arguments or outbursts of anger often stem from a lack of awareness of your mind-set. In such circumstances, you allow your emotions to overcome your confidence, calmness, and ability to make a joke out of the situation. Caught up in frustration or exasperation, you become a prisoner to your emotions. Instead of mindfully addressing the situation—calming yourself down and inserting a bit of tactful humor—you tense up, become defensive, and derail your ability to make good decisions.

While most visible in highly charged situations, a lack of awareness takes its toll on your day-to-day effectiveness as well. Looking back over a long, hectic day, you may see that you've been needlessly uptight or grave; or that you allowed a disappointing setback to upset you and ruin your productivity for the rest of the day; or that while you did an adequate job demonstrating your services to potential clients, you didn't really show them a good time, or meld the type of relationship in which they are actually excited about your next meeting. While heated moments demand vigilant awareness, sometimes it's more difficult to remain alert to your energy and emotions throughout the course of ordinary events.

Enhancing your awareness of your state of mind enables you to deal more effectively with any situation by allowing you to exercise greater control over your thoughts and emotions. Awareness limbers up the mind. It creates the resilience to absorb anxiety, and the flexibility to turn complicated problems into enticing opportunities. Attuned to your internal state, you can harness anger or tension in volatile situations. Mindful of your thinking processes, you can free yourself of rigid, limiting beliefs and concentrate your mind on challenges with soaring levels of enthusiasm and imagination. Heightened self-awareness leads to heightened self-mastery.

Self-awareness, essentially, is the art of observing your mind. It requires you to withdraw to a less involved point, and passively witness the thoughts, perceptions, and feelings traversing through your brain. The emphasis is on your position as observer. For example, when you're aware of your state of mind, you don't "feel angry"; you notice, with calm detachment, that you are experiencing the feeling of anger. As your boss is announcing impossible deadlines for your project, you don't get anxious; you tranquilly note a feeling of tension. The difference may seem subtle, but its consequences can be substantial: when you're aware of your mind-set, you see more options and remain in control.

I always use such a dualistic perspective when I'm onstage giving a presentation. Knowing that the delivery is as important as the message itself, I've learned to "stand behind myself" as I speak. Observing the details of my performance as I'm intently discussing various aspects of business and biochemistry with the audience, I notice that I need to raise my excitement level a notch, or that I'm slightly concerned about the time remaining, or other details about my voice, posture, and style. Acting as my own coach, I spur myself on: "You're feeling a little too staid, time to lighten things up with a joke, you're doing great now. . . ." Maintaining such a constant awareness of my mind and performance is invaluable to staying in top form throughout the presentation.

Anyone familiar with meditation knows the process of paying attention to your mind. Henepola Gunaratana, in an excellent description of mindfulness meditation in his book *Mindfulness,* puts it like this: "We learn to watch the arising of thought and perception with a feeling of serene detachment. We learn to view our own reactions to stimuli with calm and clarity. We begin to see ourselves reacting without getting caught up in the reactions themselves." In case that seems excessively cerebral, let me emphasize that it is a very practical technique. Employed skillfully, it can help you bypass anxiety and frustration, stop your runaway thoughts, and consciously focus your thinking where it proves most productive.

Increasing Awareness of Stressful Times

Further, becoming aware of your reactions to specific stress-inducing events radically improves your ability to effectively cope with difficult situations. If you've got a big deadline coming up or a particularly difficult week, then you've got to carefully adhere to a regimen that maximizes your energy and resilience. People often use periods of urgency as an excuse to abandon healthy habits. Of course, your reaction should be precisely the opposite: throughout the strenuous stretch, whether it is a pressure-cooker afternoon or a crucial final quarter, you have to *increase* your commitment to your energy-optimizing diet and exercise program. You have to set aside and vigilantly guard a couple of short intervals in the day in which you can meaningfully relax yourself. (As busy as I know many people are, I think there are exceptionally few individuals who are so tied up that they can't fit in two 5-minute sessions a day to stretch, breathe deeply, or go for a walk.) And you have to constantly stay attuned to your emotions and anxiety levels, maintaining optimistic self-talk and reminding yourself to see the levity inherent in even the most stressful deals.

The idea applies, as well, to specific situations or events that evoke fear, rigidity, or overzealous earnestness. Most people have one or two responsibilities that seem to summon to the surface everything about them that is low and mean. Maybe it's a bi-weekly, one-on-one meeting with your manager, or perhaps a quarterly presentation that you have to give to the rest of the staff. Whatever it is (and you should think this through—which few obligations cause you the most grief?), becoming aware of its impact on you enables you to specially prepare yourself for it.

Gretchen Shine, General Manager of Cox Cable in Roanoke, Virginia, knows perfectly well which situation tends to set her on edge. "I have to meet with governmental officials for meetings in which we're on opposing sides of a very important issue," Shine says. Fully aware of the nature of the beast (the meeting, not the government), she has a ritual rehearsal for the encounter. "In addition to being very prepared," Shine says, "I shut my door for ten minutes before I leave to have a period of quiet time to myself." During this time, she focuses and assures herself: "I try to antici-pate what the worst question would be that could possibly come up, and prepare myself for that. I talk to myself in a positive way— 'You're prepared, you know what you need to convey; they're probably going to accept part of it, not all of it,' and so on." Paying attention to the times that put your energy and patience on trial— and then taking steps to help you maintain your optimal state of mind throughout the interval—enables you to exercise greater control, build confidence, and perform at your highest level.

Optimizing Your Optimism

Almost anyone who has achieved success—as the likes of Hewlett, Packard, Honda, and Smith attest—has also achieved a great number of failures. For pioneers and inventors, it is almost axiomatic: in the course of your work, you will inevitably encounter frustration and fiasco. Honda was almost proud of his defeats. As he said in a classic speech when accepting an honorary doctorate in Michigan, "Many people dream of success. To me success can be achieved only through repeated failure and introspection. In fact, success represents the 1 percent of your work that results from the 99 percent that is called failure."

The key to triumphing over setbacks and defeat is a sense of optimism. Some people picture optimists as happy-go-lucky simpletons who frolic in unreality. But optimism doesn't refer to naive idealism. The attitude refers to a confident state of mind, the belief that you can succeed, and the expectation that your actions will produce the intended results. The practice of optimism involves focusing on the reassuring, encouraging, and hopeful elements of a situation. It is the opposite of becoming depressed, overwhelmed, or discouraged. And it is essential to persist through the part of your work called failure to produce the part called success.

Like other mental attitudes, optimism can be learned and developed. Recent work by Martin Seligman, Professor of Psychology at the University of Pennsylvania and the author of *Learned Optimism,* offers intriguing new evidence on how you can build this positive mentality into your emotional disposition. Other strategies allow you to maintain your confidence despite discouraging circumstances. By learning some of these ways of thinking about your challenges, and especially about your failures, you can develop your ability to persist through setbacks and perform optimally in the face of defeat.

A good deal of research on the connection between self-talk, optimism, persistence, and success demonstrates the powerful effect of your thinking and self-talk on performance. Some of the most interesting studies were conducted with Martin Seligman and MetLife Insurance Company, where Seligman worked with insurance salespeople for several years. Selling insurance is discouraging work, with towering rates of rejection. (Most people don't like spending a lot of money for something they can't see and

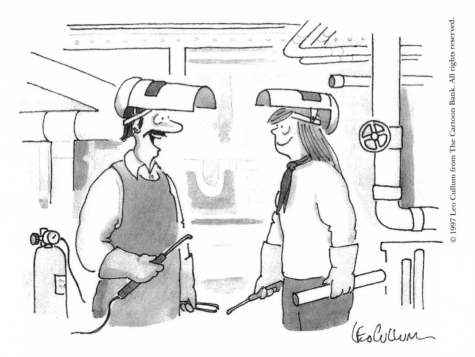

"Does it get any better than this, Melody? We're young. We're in love. And we're welders!"

rarely use, and they don't look forward to meeting someone trying to convince them to do so. "We're looked at as the human embodiment of a flu shot," says Kyle Duffold, who owns an insurance company in Colorado.) Because of the discouraging nature of the job, about three-quarters of salespeople quit in their first three years.

To find out if optimism affected job performance, Seligman and MetLife conducted some experiments, the results of which were quite revealing. In one experiment, new salespeople who were by nature optimists outsold those who were not by a remarkable 37 percent. In a second experiment, a special group of applicants who failed MetLife's normal screening tests but scored high on a test of optimism were compared to a group who passed the screening test but rated low on the optimism scale. The special optimistic group sold 21 percent more insurance their first year and 57 percent more in their second year—persuasive evidence of the power of optimism.

So how do you beef up your optimism? Maintaining positive expectations is the overriding ability, but two specific tools can help. Transforming your self-talk from a pessimistic conversation to a positive, confident dialogue helps you stay optimistic. In fact, such talk not only changes your mind-set but also makes physical changes in your body. Additionally, visualizing your goal can supply a source of optimism when you can't seem to see around the obstacles in front of you. Discouragement often attacks when you've forgotten why you are working so hard; recalling a vibrant image of achieving your goal solidifies your sense of purpose and resolve.

Telling Yourself a Good Story

After years of research, Seligman found that the single best predictor of optimism was how people talked to themselves after experiencing a setback or failure. From this new evidence comes the key strategy for persistence: changing negative internal dialogue to hopeful, reassuring, or humorous conversation.

We all talk to ourselves continually throughout the day. We comment on our appearance, critique our actions, and tell ourselves that we should do this or that. And more than most people imagine, this internal talk shapes our feelings and beliefs, which in turn affect both our physiology and our ability to perform. The reason this is so important is that most people's self-talk is negative, overly critical, and unrealistically pessimistic. Most people, in other words, are continually undermining their confidence, their positive expectations, and even their physical health by the perpetual negative dialogue that runs through their minds. Recognizing and changing these internal conversations to a more optimistic tone can help you transform your mind-set.

Marty Paradise, General Manager of Microsoft's southeastern region, feels that monitoring your self-talk substantially affects your mood and performance. Paradise says that he has been around many people who had a habit of voicing their problems and complaints until they had left themselves thoroughly discouraged: "I've seen a lot of people talk themselves into a bad mood."

Highly aware of such pitfalls, Paradise exorcises negative and self-limiting vocabulary from his speech. "I never leave the programming of my mind to chance—I consciously program it daily with specific positive directives." In fact, Paradise uses affirmations and his mission statement to direct his thoughts toward his desired goals. "I learned at an early age that I could change my performance by changing my thinking."

Self-talk is particularly important when interpreting failures. Studies show that what you say to yourself after a defeat—a project that runs aground or a missed promotion—is a crucial determinant of your ability to maintain a positive mind-set and persist through difficult situations. After meeting with rejection, pessimists get discouraged, telling themselves that they are no good, that they will never be any good, and that their life is going nowhere. Optimists, on the other hand, take defeat in stride. They tell themselves that external circumstances caused their failure and they will do better next time.

One such optimistic person is Tom McQuillan, a general agent of Canada Life and President of McQuillan Life Insurance Agencies in Toronto, and one of only twenty-five people in the world who have qualified twenty years in a row for "Top of the Table," the elite of the elite in the insurance industry. McQuillan says he has absolutely no "phone reluctance" (in fact, Canada Bell awarded him a free phone because he runs up one of the fifty highest phone bills in Canada) because he thinks through his phone calls until he feels comfortable with why his prospects need him. He visualizes the customer and his or her financial needs, and rehearses the details of his upcoming conversation in his mind. "Nothing can be lost through an intelligent approach regarding why the potential client should see me," McQuillan says. "Once I'm convinced a prospect needs me, I look forward to the call. I consider each call an investment, which is why I plan so conscientiously and fully expect to get an appointment." If his call ends without an appointment or even a pleasant response, McQuillan responds like a consummate optimist: "It must have been a bad day for the guy, so I'll call back until I get him on a good day."

We all reproach ourselves on occasion. But whether it's a rare occurrence or a habitual pattern, you have to transform the pessimistic talk that sows the seeds of discouragement to more optimistic discussion. The first step is to begin to consciously listen to the conversations you have with yourself, especially those just after a setback of some sort. Then it's a matter of deliberately replacing the negative talk ("I'm no good at this; I'll never make it") with more hopeful dialogue ("I'll have to try a different approach; the next one is mine"). Making better conversation with yourself in this way creates the optimism and persistence that allow you to perform at your highest levels, even if you're under the gun.

Visualization

On waking up each morning, Barry Triller, Executive Vice President of Mutual Life of Canada, goes through a simple visualization. "I literally picture something that will be interesting—something in the day that is going to be challenging and exciting," Triller says. The image motivates him to attack the day in a fun, optimistic frame of mind, even if his schedule promises to be hectic. "No matter what else is going on," Triller says, "I know I've got something to look forward to, something exciting to do."

Whether you are making progress toward a clearly established goal, or stuck in a rut of fatigue or frustration, visualizing a desired future state or event—an outrageously great product, a smoothly functioning store, a successful sales presentation—is another exceptional way to inspire optimistic thinking. The strategy conjures up the positive attitudes and feelings of a triumphant situation, and allows you to work in that frame of mind right now. Additionally, visualizing the future state reminds you of what you are working for and why you are doing it. It affords you a renewed sense of optimism and inspiration, and allows you to keep your current problems in perspective.

The practice of visualization has many valuable applications. Many professional athletes have made it a staple in their training programs, dedicating as much as two hours a day to envisioning themselves in action—executing the perfect dive, hitting the ball out of the park, receiving the gold medal. The power of visualization stems from the fact that the brain thinks, most fundamentally, in pictures. And the pictures that you bring to mind, either consciously or unconsciously, affect your physiology and your thinking. So physiologically, when you picture yourself calmly, confidently negotiating a difficult contract or a sales demonstration, it changes your body's chemistry to a more relaxed, self-assured state. On a psychological level, it helps you feel the emotions of the future moment.

One good practice involves visualizing the person you eventually want to be in life, with as many vivid details as possible. Where will you be? What will you be doing? Who will be with you? What will you be wearing? How will you be conducting yourself? Another great use for short-term motivation is to picture the triumphant realization of a short-term goal. Again, with as many details as possible, see yourself successfully accomplishing the project or landing the contract. Visualizing a desired state gives you an enhanced sense of confidence and a greater motivation to achieve it.

Wake Up and Take Charge of Your Mind

By paying more attention to and changing your thoughts with such tools as optimistic self-talk and visualization, you can create an optimistic mind-set and ignite top performance. To reemphasize, most people, aided by a fast-paced, high-pressure business environment, undermine themselves with negative talk and pessimistic thinking. But performing at your best requires that you take control of your mind. In order to handle difficult setbacks, energize your team, and boldly create new products and markets, you have to rid yourself of such pessimism and cultivate an excited, optimistic state of mind.

William James, one of America's preeminent psychologists and philosophers, was a devoted believer in the transformative capacities of the human mind. As James said, "It is only by risking ourselves from one hour to another that we live at all. And often enough our faith beforehand in an uncertified result is the only thing that makes the result come true."

CATCHFIRE TIPS TO MASTER YOUR MIND

1. *Tune in to your mind-set throughout the day.* Observe your state of mind four or five times during the day. How's your energy? What state are you in?
2. *Focus on your breathing.* Take slower, deeper breaths to instill a sense of calmness and confidence.
3. *Check your posture.* Straighten out the crook in your back and assume the bearing of a fearless marine. Turn your walk into a stride.
4. *Pay more attention to what you eat.* Various foods and drinks affect your mind-set. How's your mood 30 minutes after drinking a large soft drink?
5. *Set a cue in the environment.* Choose a picture, the arrival of the mail, something on your desk that can prompt you to refocus yourself. Dan Robertson of the Printing Industries of America has a screen saver on his computer that prompts him to adopt a more mindful attitude.
6. *Monitor your internal dialogue.* When you hear yourself blaming and criticizing yourself, stop! As Paul Violassi of Softech Solutions says, "Get your mind out of the gutter."
7. *Watch your self-talk.* Rephrase negative self-talk in a more hopeful, humorous manner.
8. *Visualize.* Recall past moments of brilliance and grace; envision yourself flourishing in difficult situations.

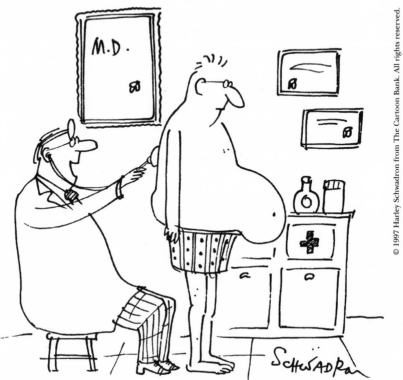

"Actually, we're finding lots of middle-management executives who can't manage their middles, Mr. Stone."

STEP 2
Eating for Performance: Food for Thought

You can manage your moods, boost your mental capabilities, and maximize your performance easily and almost instantly by eating foods that have the desired effect on the chemistry of your brain.
　　—Judith Wurtman, *Managing Your Mind and Mood Through Food*

Many companies I give presentations to immediately implement one of the simple changes I recommend: ridding their offices of the scourge of doughnuts, and replacing them with bagels (with little or no cream cheese or butter) and fruit. In some organizations, substituting the glazed and sprinkled rings with a variety of fresh fruit has become protocol—each staff meeting or company-wide conference starts off with a collective munching of apples, bananas, and oranges. Several companies have even written a fruit expense into the budget, having a supply delivered daily to their cafeteria or reception area for everyone to enjoy throughout the day.

What's the big deal about pastries and fruit? Like all foods, doughnuts and apples change the chemistry of your body and brain in a way that affects your ability to think and perform. Doughnuts, while traditional fare in meeting rooms across the nation, are deep-fried, heavily sweetened circles of dough that possess enough fat and sugar to derail constructive thinking and deaden the collective spirit of a gathering. Fruit, on the other hand, provides a natural, steady source of energy that sparks inventive thinking and productive work sessions.

Beyond the physiological effects of these foods, the difference strikes me as symbolic. Meetings that feature boxes of chocolate-covered, cheese-stuffed, jelly-filled items seem to drag, as if the thick ooze of the pastries somehow bogs down the discussion and ideas. Groups gathered around a tray of fresh fruit, by contrast, usually seem stimulating and enthusiastic—almost as if the freshness and crispness carry over into the conversation and planning. People who adopt the custom invariably tell me that serving fruit sets a new, energetic tone for their discussions. "We have an unspoken rule that we have no afternoon meeting without fruit," says John Leavitt of the Health Care Initiative, Inc. "As a result, people stay awake and alert. Fruit brings you alive."

Eating Strategically

You've undoubtedly heard about the effects of eating habits on your health. Regularly eating foods laden with fat, cholesterol, sugar, and preservatives can clog your arteries, make you fat, suppress your immune system, and deny your body the essential nutrients it needs to function well. When consumed in excess, foods such as doughnuts, candy bars, hot dogs, and fried chicken can contribute to cardiovascular disease, obesity, diabetes, and certain forms of cancer. A nutritious diet, on the other hand, enhances the overall functioning of your system. Eating a low-fat diet that includes plenty of fruits, vegetables, and grains supplies your body with the building blocks to synthesize healthy skin, muscles, organs, and bones.

But more than preventing illness, eating the right foods at the right times—eating strategically, Step 2 of the CatchFire program—optimizes your energy, mood, and ability to perform on the job. Eating strategically consists of following a few fairly simple guidelines, such as eating less fat and refined sugar, breaking up three large meals into five or six smaller ones (by simply reducing the size of your regular meals and adding a couple of healthy snacks), eating certain foods at lunch to energize your system throughout the afternoon, and taking moderate-dose vitamin supplements to ensure that your body is getting all the nutrients it needs. Over the long run, such eating habits help maintain your general health and vitality. More immediately, eating certain foods can reduce tension and mood swings, increase energy and alertness, and put you into the state in which you work at your best.

All foods are drugs. Every bagel, carrot, or hamburger you chew and swallow changes the chemistry of your body and brain. And while the effects of a Big Mac are less spectacular than the effects of, say, cocaine, all foods produce physiological alterations that enhance or detract from your ability to put together a quality report or pull off a brilliant presentation. Aside from nourishing the systems that sustain energy and well-being, your eating habits have an immediate impact on your biochemistry in two other important ways.

Your food intake changes your blood sugar level. A normal blood sugar level—maintained by eating frequently and eating complex carbohydrates—keeps a steady flow of glucose to the brain (which depends solely on glucose and oxygen as its sources of energy), and thereby promotes consistent energy levels and stable, positive moods. Rapid jumps and declines in blood sugar levels—caused predominantly by skipping meals or by consuming food or drink with high concentrations of refined sugar—often lead to fatigue, nervousness, and irritability.

Additionally, certain foods adjust the chemical balance in the brain in a way that modifies your energy and mood. Recent research led by Judith Wurtman, Ph.D., of the Massachusetts Institute of Technology, demonstrates how eating carbohydrates—such as a bagel, low-fat muffin, or bag of pretzels—can increase the presence of serotonin in the brain, a chemical that has a calming, tension-relieving, focusing effect. Additionally, studies show that eating protein—such as chicken, fish, or very lean beef—triggers an influx of the "alertness chemicals" dopamine and norepinephrine, which raises your energy and drive. Knowing how to use these foods to your advantage equips you with an outstanding tool to maximize your mental capacities.

(Sometimes the idea of "adjusting your brain chemistry" raises alarm. By way of reassurance, all of the recommendations in this chapter are perfectly safe. They involve, quite simply, the occasional substitution of one common food for another, or taking widely prescribed, moderate-dose vitamin supplements. To reemphasize, we're made of chemicals, and anytime you get angry, laugh, go for a jog, or eat a sandwich, you alter your brain chemistry. The goal is to produce healthy alterations that enhance your mental performance.)

The point is you can stumble through the day dull and drowsy because you deprive yourself of the foods that adequately fuel your body and brain. Or you can charge through your day (taking time for a couple of short breaks) with an energetic, focused mind-set because you fortify yourself with powerpacked meals. Many people overlook the connection between their diet and their productivity. But if you're a salesperson, your energy and emotions are just as important as your product. If you're a manager, your ability to inspire your team to implement a plan is just as important as having the right plan. Whatever your position, you need to take a well-nourished brain to work just as surely as you need to take your briefcase.

Are You Fit for Top Performance?

To get an idea about your current fitness level—or how well you are preparing yourself to work productively—take the following Fitness Profile to discover the quality of your health habits. The quiz covers information in this and upcoming chapters, and it will give you valuable feedback about what changes you can make to boost your ability to perform.

FITNESS PROFILE

	Always	Often	Sometimes	Seldom	Never
I eat something healthy for breakfast daily.	5	4	3	2	1
I eat 4 to 5 smaller meals daily.	5	4	3	2	1
I eat fruit and vegetables daily.	5	4	3	2	1
Less than 30% of my daily caloric intake is fat.	5	4	3	2	1
I take vitamin supplements daily.	5	4	3	2	1
I eat fried foods daily.	1	2	3	4	5
I eat red meat daily.	1	2	3	4	5
I drink 6 to 8 glasses of water daily.	5	4	3	2	1
I monitor my sugar intake.	5	4	3	2	1
I have more than two alcoholic drinks daily.	1	2	3	4	5
I exercise aerobically at least 3 times a week.	10	8	3	2	1
I exercise with weights or Nautilus-type machines 2 times per week.	5	4	3	2	1
I take breaks 2 times per day in addition to lunch.	5	4	3	2	1
I sleep 7 or 8 hours per night.	5	4	3	2	1
I actively cultivate relationships and interests outside of work.	5	4	3	2	1
I laugh 20 or more times per day.	5	4	3	2	1
I take adequate time off for vacations.	5	4	3	2	1
I practice a relaxation technique daily.	5	4	3	2	1
My energy level is high.	5	4	3	2	1
TOTALS					

To score your Fitness Profile, add the numbers you have circled. The total is your score.

80–100	Excellent Health Habits	Total Score _____
70–79	Good Health Habits	
60–69	Special Attention	
59 & below	Red Alert!!	

Nutrients of Performance

Gallup polls conducted over the last ten years indicate that more and more people have a concept of health that doesn't revolve around avoiding illness or living to age 90 as much as it centers on performing at their best. The Professional Workforce Survey paralleled those findings. As the survey showed, most business-people view their food choices—whether they order a hamburger and fries at lunch or choose the turkey sandwich—as more than a way to stave off distant heart attacks. In fact, about *three-fourths* of the respondents believe that their food intake significantly influences their energy level, attitude, and ability to perform at work (53 percent said that their diet is "very important" to their energy level). A comparison of those who regularly snack at the salad bar to those who frequently visit the vending machines reveals a convincing correlation between a healthy diet and on-the-job effectiveness.

In the survey, people who rated themselves as having excellent eating habits had a more positive attitude about their jobs than those with poor eating habits, and more often reported themselves to be top performers at work. Additionally, there was a pronounced difference in tension levels between healthy eaters and junk-food junkies. Perhaps because of the fatigue and nervousness that can result from eating sugary foods, people with poor eating habits were more than twice as likely to feel that they were under heavy stress. By contrast, professionals with excellent eating habits were significantly less likely to get frustrated or anxious in the face of problems.

Almost all of the people I interviewed echoed the feeling that eating well improves attitude and productivity. While some reported only a subtle effect, many were emphatic in their endorsement of the benefits of a high-energy diet. Jodi Hobbs, a marketing specialist with Microsoft, is one who finds her food choices to have a potent effect on her energy and enthusiasm. She recently converted to healthier eating habits primarily to improve her physical health, but found that the changes also sparked an upsurge in her energy level. "A few months ago I started on a very big health kick as far as my eating goes," Hobbs says. "I can't believe how much more energy I have now—more than I've ever had before. I can't even tell you what a difference it has made." (And Microsoft makes it easy for her to know what to choose. Like other enlightened companies I've worked with, Microsoft labels the nutritional breakdown of all the food in their campus eateries. In fact, when I was visiting their headquarters in Redmond, Washington, one of the cafeterias had a sign under the pastries that read "Eat these and die.")

Jim Ruybal of United Artists also believes a healthy diet is a key component of consistently feeling great and maintaining high productivity. While Ruybal eats healthy foods all day long, his lunchtime regimen is particularly important, when he takes an hour and a half to work out, shower, and eat a light, nutritious lunch. The one-two punch of a workout and healthy lunch completely revitalizes his energy and perspective: "I can leave with a stack of messages and problems on my desk, and come back an hour and a half later, and they don't look so insurmountable. I grab the tough messages and decide to call them back right away." Ruybal says the energy boost seems especially advantageous when compared to the mild stupor that most people experience after lunch. "I usually have a salad after I work out," he says. "I go into meetings and everyone else has just had a big lunch. They're bogged down, and I'm ready to go."

Dietary Misconceptions

Although a wide majority of people believes that eating healthy foods significantly affects their performance, many people say that their diet leaves considerable room for improvement. On a scale of 1 to 10, most of the professionals in the Professional Workforce Survey rated their eating habits at about 6—a score I equate with a "D." What's stopping them from eating smarter? Time is a big factor. If you're grabbing a bite on the way to work or between meetings, many of your choices—fast-food restaurants, convenience stores, or vending machines—are occupied by a standing army of sugar and fat. But for most people, poor eating habits stem from a combination of not wanting to restrict themselves to a diet of "health food" and simply not knowing enough about how various foods affect them.

Fortunately, these obstacles are not difficult to overcome. With an upgrade in your nutritional knowledge and awareness, you can adopt a diet that enhances your energy and mood, and still satisfies your desire for enjoyable food. This chapter provides a solid overview, but taking an active interest in health articles, food labels, and food preparation will quickly establish you as a capable judge of which foods will sharpen your focus and which will dull your mind. As you learn and experiment, you'll find countless recipes and entrées that meet the dual standards for taste and nutrition. And you'll provide yourself the fuel to power through long days of productive activity.

While many people who regularly feed at the fast-food trough will have some substantial modifications to make, eating health-fully doesn't mean eating like a Puritan or a prude. You don't have to meticulously count calories or stock up on bran flakes and tofu. In addition to dining on abundant portions of fresh fruits and vegetables, whole-grain breads, potatoes, rice, and beans in various delectable preparations, you can selectively indulge your craving for a preposterously high-fat cut of beef, slice of cheesecake, or ice cream sundae. The fundamental goal is not to lose twenty pounds in a month, but to sustain healthful habits for the rest of your life. And in fact, most people who learn to order or prepare more fresh, low-fat foods and adopt a more mindful style of eating not only feel more energetic but also find that they derive more satisfaction from their meals.

Eating Through the Ages

Various tribes and civilizations throughout history have lived on extremely different diets. Some Eskimo tribes consumed pre-dominantly high-fat, animal-based foods. Many Asian populations prospered on a diet consisting primarily of rice and vegetables. As such a wide diversity attests, the human body is remarkably adaptable and resilient, and can survive on a great variety of energy sources.

Nonetheless, our species didn't evolve to function optimally on many of the foods that make up the common diet. In fact, anthropologists believe that for the vast majority of humankind's time on earth, our ancestors subsisted mainly on complex carbohydrates like grains, berries, fruits, and vegetables. The immense quantities of processed food that make up the bulk of the typical American diet—complete with large amounts of fat, sugar, sodium, and other preservatives—constitute a major deviation from our formerly high-carbohydrate sustenance. And it causes a shock to our system. Particularly jolting is the massively increased intake of refined sugar. The average American ingests approximately 127 pounds of the stuff per year, compared to about a *tenth* of that for the average person in the nineteenth century. As I'll discuss shortly, this influx can create a serious imbalance in mind and mood.

Many experts think these drastic dietary changes, combined with a sharp decrease in physical activity, contribute to many of the illnesses (such as heart disease) that afflict our civilization. At the very least, they prevent our bodies from getting the dietary fuel—predominantly natural complex carbohydrates—on which they were designed to function optimally.

Food Fundamentals

On a very basic level, healthy eating habits enhance your ability to perform by keeping your physiological systems in good shape. All the organs, glands, nerves, and neurotransmitters that work together to create a state of energy and focus—the enthusiasm necessary to motivate your team or convince your boss to adopt a new idea of yours—are built from and powered by the foods you eat (and to some extent, from the oxygen you breathe). When you eat foods that supply your body with the nutrients it needs,

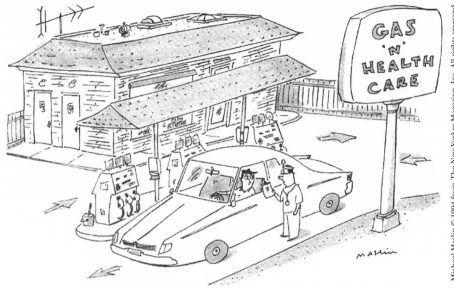

"Your oil's fine, but your blood sugar level's a little low."

you help these millions of complex processes run efficiently. As a result, your body and brain stay vital and vigorous.

Eating an unhealthy diet, on the other hand, can cause a variety of nutritional deficiencies that may lead to mood-depressing chemical imbalances. Not getting enough essential nutrients (by steadfastly ignoring fruits and vegetables), for instance, can hinder your ability to productively respond to stressful situations. The overconsumption of fat is another example. Eating too much fat makes you fat. And all considerations of self-image aside, when you're storing an excessive amount of body fat, you generally don't handle stress as effectively, feel as energetic, or think as sharply.

Stabilizing Blood Sugar for Emotional Control

As just mentioned, a critical mechanism through which food affects your thinking and performance is your blood sugar level. Cells throughout your body draw on glucose in the bloodstream as their most ready source of energy. Some of them, most notably the cells in your brain, feed *only* on glucose (or more accurately, glu-cose from the food you eat and oxygen from the air you breathe). In fact, the brain is a glucose hog, sucking up a hefty percentage of all the glucose in your body to perform its complex processes.

When your blood sugar level is stable, you deliver ample amounts of energy to your body. Your physiological systems are well fed and happy, your brain has fuel to work through intricate business decisions, and you generally feel calm. And you can fo-cus your thoughts in a single-minded, deliberate, highly produc-tive way. (Focus is a capacity closely intertwined with blood sugar levels.) When blood sugar runs low, however, your body goes into a minor state of panic. Because glucose is the sole nourisher of the brain, your system interprets a scarcity of it as an emergency. As hypoglycemics (people who are unable to maintain adequate blood sugar) well know, you begin to feel nervous, fatigued, and irritable. Your ability to focus on your work or deal with other people evaporates, and the quality of your work takes a nosedive.

Many people trigger low blood sugar levels and the consequent negative emotions by their eating habits. Or their fasting habits, as the case may be—skipping meals is one of the most common ways to induce a glucose deficit. Rushing into a morning meeting without breakfast, toiling into the afternoon without lunch, or denying yourself snacks throughout the day prevents you from replenishing the glucose in your system. And as it runs down, so does your enthusiasm, focus, and patience.

Ingesting a heavy dose of refined white sugar is another way to induce low blood sugar levels. A surprising reaction on the sur-face (how does eating sugar decrease blood sugar?), this response should convert anyone who reaches for a candy bar as a pick-me-up. As researchers have found, eating a sugar snack gives you a quick shot of vitality that is soon followed by a state of decreased energy, increased tension, and scattered focus—a brief lift-off fol-lowed by a crash landing. Here's what happens physiologically: The simple sugar (or sucrose) of the soft drink or candy bar is rapidly absorbed into the bloodstream—too rapidly, in fact (re-member that our systems didn't evolve to digest such refined forms of sugar). Your blood sugar shoots up to unacceptably high levels, and to counter the overabundance, the pancreas secretes the hormone insulin, which pushes the glucose out of the blood-stream and into the body's muscle cells. Fifteen minutes to an hour after eating the sugary food, your blood sugar is much lower than it was before you ate the snack, and your brain is left scrambling for fuel.

The best way to maintain adequate blood sugar levels is simply to counter these habits by eating often and avoiding foods with refined sugar. Instead of soft drinks (which contain an average of ten teaspoons of sugar) and candy, choose fruit, bagels, low-salt pretzels, low-fat popcorn, or low-fat granola bars. And while you shouldn't snack with abandon, eating light, healthy snacks mid-morning and midafternoon maintains a strong, constant fuel source. Paul Violassi of Softech Solutions is one of many who have found that such eating habits produce a major difference in energy and attitude. "I used to suffer from being real tired at ten in the morning, going into a food coma just after lunch, and getting real tired at about three in the afternoon," says Violassi. "I don't have that problem at all anymore, and I think eating the right foods during the day helped a lot. I stay away from processed sugars. I eat three to five pieces of fruit a day, and I've got a bag of carrots at my desk. It keeps the energy up—I feel great."

Eating frequently, in fact, proves to be a remarkably valuable tool for consistently maintaining the blood sugar levels that promote energy, focus, and calmness. Research has repeatedly shown that consuming your foods in smaller, lighter meals helps ward off frustration and anxiety, and encourages a more steady, energetic frame of mind. Dr. David Jenkins of the University of Toronto conducted one of the more dramatic experiments on this topic. In his experiment, two groups were fed identical diets but consumed their food on different eating schedules: the first group had three relatively large meals and the second group had seventeen small meals over the day. After two weeks, those on the "nibbling diet" had a remarkable 15 percent reduction in blood cholesterol, 17 percent reduction in cortisol (a hormone associated with the feeling of negative stress), and 28 percent reduction in insulin (high levels of insulin indicate unbalanced blood sugar levels and therefore greater instability of emotions and energy levels). Eating seventeen times a day, to be sure, isn't necessary. Eating five or six times confers nearly the same advantages (and you don't have to keep your pockets filled with food).

Powerful Proteins and Calming Carbohydrates

A final way that foods influence your performance involves the effects that protein and carbohydrates have on the chemistry of your brain. While useful articles and books have been published on the subject, very few businesspeople make use of this practical, effective way to calm a scattered mind or ignite energy and alertness.

Dr. Judith Wurtman at M.I.T. has pioneered much of the research in this area. Many of her studies consist of feeding groups of people different meals and then testing them, using a variety of different measurements, on their energy level, mood, and performance. In the experiments, a group of people fill out questionnaires that pinpoint their mood states. Then each person is given a meal—some get a "calming" meal, others get an "energizing" meal. After eating, the subjects fill out mood surveys once an hour for three hours. How did they rate themselves?

As Wurtman reports, "Those who eat the calming foods consistently report feeling more relaxed, more focused, less stressed, less distracted after their meal." In addition to their testimony, their performance on behavioral tests showed them to be relaxed and focused. Eating "energizing" food, Wurtman says, produces equally significant results: "Those who eat the energizing foods report feeling more alert and motivated after their meal, and *their* performance tests show speedier responses and increased accuracy."

The physiological changes underlying these shifts in energy

and mood involve the effect of carbohydrates (the calming food) and protein (the energizing food) on the levels of different neurotransmitters in your brain. Consuming carbohydrates causes a relatively greater incidence of the amino acid tryptophan in the bloodstream, which stimulates the production of the neurotransmitter serotonin—a chemical that has a calming effect on your mood. Eating protein, on the other hand, blocks the entry of tryptophan into the brain, thereby preventing serotonin and its mellowing effect. And further, protein increases the level of the amino acid tyrosine in the bloodstream, which encourages the brain to make more of the neurotransmitters dopamine and norepinephrine—chemicals that produce a boost in energy and alertness.

You can make use of these effects anytime you eat. The most useful application of this "eating strategy," for many people, is to eat more protein at lunch and thereby work with greater energy and zest throughout the second part of the day. If you've got a big afternoon in front of you, stay away from the pasta and choose a turkey sandwich or a chicken, fish, or lean beef entrée. (As for portion size, a good rule of thumb is that your meat or fish should be about as big as a deck of cards if you're having it as an entrée, or about half as much for a snack.) On the other hand, when you're feeling frazzled during a session of intense meetings, snack on complex carbohydrates to help you relax and focus.

The following are some of the best foods to trigger these respective responses. (Fruits and vegetables are excellent foods—they're packed with nutrients and help maintain stable moods by supplying a steady source of blood sugar. But these foods are broken down too slowly to significantly alter brain biochemistry, and therefore they don't activate either the calm or energetic effect.)

Powerful Proteins	*Calming Carbohydrates*
Low-fat meats	Bread and bagels
Fish	Pasta
Bean soups and salads	Low-fat crackers
Low-fat yogurt	Low-fat muffins

Powerful Proteins	*Calming Carbohydrates*
Low-fat cottage cheese	Dry cereal
Tofu	Oatmeal
Chicken	Potatoes
Turkey	Rice

Adopting a High-Performance Diet

Thriving in today's business world requires peak levels of physical stamina and the mental capacity to smoothly handle change and adversity. It demands that you think of yourself as a performer—like an athlete approaching the playing field. And like an athlete, you have to strategically approach your lifestyle—including your eating habits—in a way that will help you stay in the energy zone.

A high-performance diet helps you maximize your physical vigor and vitality, and attack problems with enhanced mental focus and alertness. Its main components are the following:

1. Eat a diet low in fat and high in complex carbohydrates, or more specifically, a diet in which calories come from approximately 65 percent carbohydrates, 15 percent protein, and 20 percent fat.
2. Graze, don't gorge; eat several (five or six) small meals and snacks throughout the day. (Reduce the size of your regular meals and add a couple of healthy snacks.)
3. Avoid refined sugar as much as possible.
4. Eat protein at lunch or at other times when you need to remain optimally alert and energized.

As with all meaningful change, you have to make good eating habits an integral part of your lifestyle. The first step toward such a goal is to shun all diets in their ordinary form—the restrictive, often weird regimens claiming that you can lose twenty pounds in a month by eating only grapefruit. Studies show that 95 percent of the people who lose weight on rigid diets gain it back, many people ending up with more pounds than they started with. In addition, most diets produce a host of unhealthy changes in your body that compromise your fitness and vitality. The only real way to improve your health, mentality, and performance is to take a lifelong approach, adopting eating habits that you will follow through the advanced years of your life (which will undoubtedly prove longer and more vigorous because of your food selections).

A second element in your strategy—an indispensable element in sustaining a lifelong commitment—is to maintain eating habits that are not only healthy but also satisfying and enjoyable. Dining is too pleasurable an activity to be reduced to staples of dry toast and cottage cheese. George Bernard Shaw may have slightly overstated the case, but he nicely captured the passion of the idea when he wrote, "There is no love sincerer than the love of food." When you learn how to buy, cook, and order healthful foods, you realize that it's not overly difficult to eat energy-boosting, performance-enhancing fare and still maintain an exciting food life.

A last parameter of eating for enhanced energy and mood is to eat more mindfully. Many rushed businesspeople have developed the habit of eating rapidly and distractedly—scarfing down their food, to put it bluntly. Surveys show that the majority of professionals often whittle down their "lunch hour" to a 30-minute period, with a significant share of these people ingesting their meal in 15 minutes or less. (The actual time spent eating, one study said, was a scant 4½ minutes.) This habit is particularly detrimental because biochemically, your stomach takes 20 minutes to signal your brain that it is full. In other words, when you eat quickly and mindlessly, you don't give yourself the chance to feel full and to decide to stop eating.

Becoming more mindful of your feeding practices—eating more slowly, chewing and tasting your food, appreciating its flavors and nourishment—helps you digest better and derive more nutritional benefit from your meals. If you can't get away for lunch with your colleagues, at least pay more attention to the sandwich you eat at your desk. Not only do you profit from increased mindfulness in enjoyment and absorption but you also

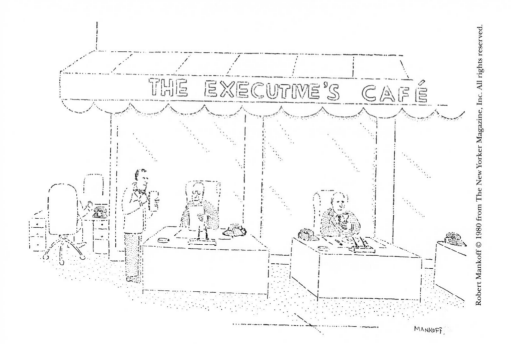

overcome the tendency to overeat. So rather than walking back from lunch feeling full and sleepy, you return to work reenergized and ready to assail your most difficult problems and projects.

The Performance Day Diet

While strategically eating protein or carbohydrate meals makes a great weapon to fend off anxiety or fatigue, your overall diet should emphasize complex carbohydrates and cut out most fat. (To repeat: the ideal diet is about 65 percent carbohydrate, 15 percent protein, and 20 percent fat.) With these guidelines in mind, base your diet around the following foods:

- *Fresh fruits*—apples, bananas, oranges, peaches, pears, grapefruit, strawberries, raspberries, blackberries, cantaloupe, watermelon, honeydew melon, pineapples, tomatoes. Fruit juices are great as well, though they aren't as good as whole fruit (they lack the fiber) and they tend to have a lot of calories.

- *Vegetables*—salads (but avoid creamy dressings, and use other dressings in moderation), potatoes, broccoli, green leaf vegetables, carrots, celery, spinach, onions, asparagus, cauliflower, beets, mushrooms, zucchini, squash, eggplant, peppers.
- *Beans and legumes*—soups, salads, or dishes featuring lentils, peas, kidney beans, white beans, black beans, split peas, soybeans, navy beans, garbanzo beans.
- *Grains*—wheat (as in bread, pasta, bagels, pita bread, pancakes), rice, corn, oats, couscous, quinoa, barley.

Eat the following foods in moderation:
- *Nonfat dairy products*—skim milk, nonfat yogurt, nonfat cheeses, egg whites.
- *Chicken*—skinless.
- *Fish*—cod, salmon, snapper, tuna, canned tuna in water, halibut, orange roughy, swordfish, flounder. Eat shellfish (shrimp, crab, lobster) less often, because they're high in cholesterol.
- *Turkey*—skinless white meat.
- *Very lean meats*—the leanest cuts of beef, buffalo, venison.

Avoid the following foods as much as possible, excluding birthdays and other festive occasions:
- *Butter, margarine, oils, and oil-containing products*—oil-based salad dressings usually have fewer calories than creamy dressings, but they are still very high in fat—use them economically.
- *High-fat dairy products*—whole milk, cream, 2 percent milk, egg yolks, yogurt (2 percent milk is not much better than whole milk—choose skim milk, or at most, 1 percent).
- *Red meats*—hamburgers, bacon, sausage, and regular (not lean) cuts of beef.
- *Fried foods.*
- *Most fast food.*
- *Sugar and simple sugar derivatives*—honey, molasses, corn syrup, high fructose corn syrup.
- *Products high in sugar or sugar derivatives*—candy, candy bars, soft drinks, most desserts.

EVERYTHING BEGINS WITH BREAKFAST

In my presentations, I always ask for a show of hands of people who don't eat breakfast. It usually amounts to half of the entire audience. Discussing the reasons behind their omission, many say they don't like to eat early or they don't have time. Few seem to consider that skipping breakfast might adversely affect their performance.

At breakfast, you literally "break" the eight- to twelve-hour "fast" since last night's dinner. The early meal is important because after several hours of not eating, your blood sugar level is low and in need of replenishment. Additionally, food in the morning "entrains" your body, enhancing biological processes and synchronizing all your body clocks and systems. In the first hour or so after awakening, your body is switching from the reduced energy expenditure, lower body temperature, and diminished hormone production of night to the more active daytime mode. Dashing out to the car without having anything to eat leaves your body and brain unfueled and untuned. As a result, you communicate less articulately in your early calls and work less productively in the morning hours.

Once you're aware of the importance of eating breakfast, you can set a strategy for starting your day with the right kind of meal. Part of the strategy is to change your attitude not just about food but also about entering another day looking for possibilities. Eating breakfast is a great way to help you learn to love the morning. A bowl of oatmeal with raisins and cinnamon can quickly convert you from a "just give me 15 more minutes" attitude to a "seize the day" mentality.

Your breakfast should be low in fat and high in complex carbohydrates. Fortunately, many appealing breakfast foods fall under those parameters. Cereals like Grape-Nuts, Wheaties, Shredded Wheat, or oatmeal are an excellent, nutrient-dense choice for your early meal. With cereal—and every time you have milk—use skim milk. Skim milk has very little fat compared to 2 percent milk, which is approximately 39 percent fat, or whole milk, which is about 50 percent fat. (The problem with skim milk, of course, is that it's blue, and blue milk in coffee or on cereal is not aesthetically pleasing. If the color violates your artistic sensibility, get $1/2$ percent or 1 percent.) Fresh fruit is another excellent choice. Cantaloupe, honeydew, grapefruit, berries, and other fruits gradually elevate blood sugar and supply you with a number of important nutrients. A fruit smoothie (provided you use low-fat or nonfat milk) makes a healthy and exciting start to the day. For those who have little time in the morning, bagels are a great breakfast item—unless you use them as cream cheese holders (though in recent years, bagels have become much bigger, supplying too many calories for some people). If you use cream cheese, choose a low-fat variety and spread it thin rather than dollop it on. Better yet, use all-fruit jelly or jam.

Jim Fitzgerald, former managing principal of Right Associates in Chicago, not only converted to regularly eating breakfast himself, but also advised his clients to do so as well. Fitzgerald's job involved helping people find and succeed in new careers. As studies show, people who lose their jobs or decide on a career change tend to lose confidence and gain weight. Fitzgerald found that by encouraging healthy eating and exercise habits, he could help people reverse this pattern and greatly aid them in their search. Starting each day with breakfast was a key component in the revamped eating habits. "Eating breakfast not only makes sense, it works," says Fitzgerald. "It has tremendous effects on your energy levels."

COFFEE

Although various studies in the past have linked caffeine intake to cancer and other serious diseases, more comprehensive recent studies haven't found any correlation between caffeine and disease in healthy individuals. But if you have a history of hypertension or heart problems, coffee might pose some risk. (Check with your doctor.)

For many people, one or two cups of coffee can pleasantly enhance mental alertness and efficiency. The brew can provide a lift in the morning, drawing you into the world of the living and making you more attentive and sharp at your early-morning breakfast meetings. But if you drink more than two 8-ounce cups (or one large cup from a coffee shop or convenience store, which is typically 16 ounces), caffeine tends to drive up feelings of nervousness and tension. The extent of this tension and the amount of caffeine required to produce it can vary greatly from one person to the next; but most people who have experienced the coffee jitters know that they make you scattered, agitated, and unproductive. If you find that you're talking a thousand words a minute and people are looking at you like you're an idiot, take it as a sign to cut back.

To be clear, caffeine is a habit-forming psychoactive drug. It stimulates your nervous system and leads to an increased amount of epinephrine and norepinephrine in your body and brain. Just as the sugar high is shortly followed by the sugar blues, coffee can cause a downturn an hour or so after you stop drinking—and therefore make you want to have another cup. So if you drink coffee, do it mindfully—have a cup to start off the day when you're feeling slow. In the long run, you're probably better off not drinking too much of it. In fact, research indicates that people who give up caffeine begin to feel more energetic after a short period of time.

I BREAK FOR FRUIT

Fruit is a perfect food to have during the midmorning and afternoon time-outs. The sugar in fruit (fructose) is *gradually* converted into glucose without the insulin response, and therefore doesn't give you the downside of refined sugar (sucrose).

Eating certain foods during your breaks can help realign your mood and energy. If you're feeling overly anxious and want to relax and concentrate, then eat carbohydrates, such as half of a bagel or some low-salt pretzels. Combined with a 5-minute deep-breathing session or a brief walk, such a snack will put you back into a more focused, composed state of mind. If you're feeling low on energy, a protein snack can help pick you up. There are many low-fat, high-protein energy bars that you can keep on hand in a desk drawer.

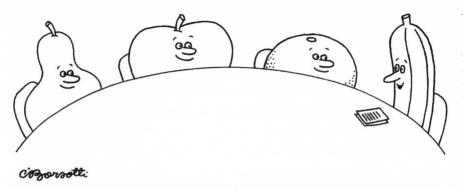

"And fruit instead of a gooey, sweet dessert is way up."

If your cafeteria is open, choose low-fat cottage cheese or a half sandwich of turkey, chicken breast, or lean roast beef.

LUNCH: LEAN AND MEAN WITH PROTEIN

The overall daily regimen for top performance on the job calls for a diet based on 65 percent carbohydrate, 20 percent fat, and 15 percent protein. Because most people experience a slump in the afternoon, a good time to eat most of that protein is at lunch.

I survey approximately twenty thousand people a year in my seminars, and 70 to 80 percent agree that mid- to late afternoon is their period of lowest energy. The American Council on Sleep, in fact, says that American business loses $15.9 billion a year in productivity between two and four o'clock in the afternoon because people are tired, unproductive, or even falling asleep at their desks.

Eating a high-protein, low-fat lunch, however, is one way to help you stay energized and alert. Your strategy for a productive afternoon should involve eating some variety of chicken, turkey, fish, lean beef, beans, legumes, or tofu. Approximately 3 to 4 ounces of protein stimulates the production of the "alertness drugs" dopamine and norepinephrine, which will keep you focused and sharp for whatever problems or decisions come your way. The one caveat is to avoid any carbohydrate—such as bread, chips, crackers, or rolls—before you eat the protein. Eating carbohydrates and proteins *at the same time* is fine, since the tyrosine will beat out the tryptophan in the race to the brain and produce the energizing effect. But eating carbohydrates first activates your body's insulin response, which automatically allows the trypto-phan to triumph and prohibits the boost in alertness.

Sandwiches with turkey breast, chicken, or very lean beef make easy, powerpacked lunches. Soups and salads that feature beans and legumes (such as split pea or lentil soup), low-fat cottage cheese, or low-fat yogurt also produce the energizing effect. An-other high-energy meal is an egg-white omelet with chicken and vegetables topped with picante sauce—a hot way to catch fire for a great afternoon of work.

ENERGY-SAPPING FOODS TO AVOID
While a double cheeseburger has a great deal of protein, this and other high-fat foods will sabotage your energy level. Eating fat shunts a large amount of blood to your digestive system—and therefore away from the brain. So, in addition to making a small contribution to your early death, fatty foods—fried foods, red meat, cream-based soups and pasta sauces, creamy salad dress-ings, cheese, a heavy coat of mayonnaise—clog your short-term thinking and slow your mental performance.

CALMING DOWN WITH DINNER
While your evening meal doesn't affect your performance as much as lunch because you're not at work, dinner is still impor-tant for your long-term energy levels and health. From a strategic point of view, dinner should help you relax from the pressures of the business day.

In the evening, a general rule is to eat more carbohydrate than protein for its ensuing calming effect. You can still have a chicken or meat dish without worrying that the protein will keep you up. But to unwind and relax, pasta with marinara or some other meatless sauce is ideal. Bread or rolls (without butter), salads, vegetables, rice, potatoes, or grains such as tabouleh or couscous are great at night. Pizza that is light on the cheese and heavy on the vegetables is great as well. As a general rule, the later the time, the lighter you eat—and try to eat at least two hours before you go to bed.

If you want dessert, a good staple is fruit. There are also many specially prepared low-calorie, low-fat desserts—such as low-fat cookies, low-fat pound cake, angel food cake—that work as satisfying, light desserts. Occasionally, of course, you have to splurge and devour a rich tiramisu or towering piece of chocolate cake. But because fat eaten at night is not usually worked off in any physical activity, you directly store it as fat tissue. In other words, you eat it, you wear it.

TO WORK AFTER DINNER, EAT PROTEIN

If you're in the midst of a project demanding late nights of work, try the following prescription: eat light, eat foods high in protein but low in fat, and eat the protein before you eat any accompanying carbohydrates. If I'm working late, I'll have a skinless breast of chicken first and then a salad or rice. As for coffee, research persuasively demonstrates that having caffeine at night interrupts sleep patterns for most of the population. If you're desperate to finish your work, drinking coffee at night will help you stay awake. But you'll very likely pay for it the next day. You shouldn't make a habit of it.

WATER

Water is almost ubiquitous, and we tend to ignore it unless thirsty. But thirst, it turns out, is no reliable way to judge dehydration or our need for water. "It's crucial to every function of the body, and even a tiny shortage can disrupt your biochemistry," says Michael Colgan, nutritional researcher and Visiting Scholar at Rockefeller University.

How much water should you drink each day? We lose 10 cups a day (not including perspiration in exercise or hard work). We gain approximately 4 cups through food. So you need 6 to 8 cups (to be on the safe side) of water per day to maintain your critical balance. Like sleep, another overlooked tool for maintaining optimal moods, water is an important variable in top performance.

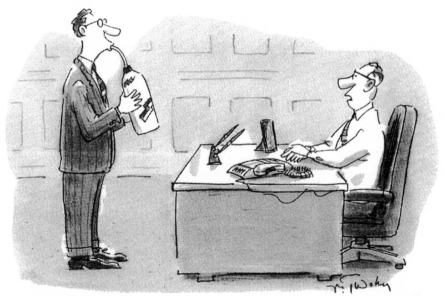

"It has come to my attention, Collins, that you are hydrating on company time."

Revitalize with Vitamins

For many years, the medical profession and many health professionals spoke of vitamin supplements as "expensive urine"—referring to the tendency of poorly manufactured products to avoid absorption and make a quick exit from the body. More recently, numerous health journals, doctors, and the American Medical Association have begun endorsing the responsible use of moderate-dose vitamin and mineral supplements, especially the antioxidant vitamins A, C, and E. Because of the toll that emotional stress, pollution, and a poor diet can take on your body, the use of vitamins and minerals, at minimum, functions as a good insurance policy. At best, it can spark energy and health. The additional nutrients can be particularly beneficial to you when you're under heavy pressure at work; in such situations, your body's nutrient needs increase and (although I urge you to continue to maintain healthy habits) you're prone to drink more coffee and eat less healthy food than usual.

Use the following guidelines when taking vitamins:

1. Take vitamins that are 100 percent natural, free of artificial colors.
2. Choose products that are nonchemically coated (with aqueous coating, for instance) and dissolve quickly in your system.
3. Take vitamins with food and water, which help absorb them more efficiently.
4. Take calcium if you're over 40, and make sure it has vitamin D in the formula.

HERBAL SUPPLEMENTS

Dietary supplements containing herbs are also becoming increasingly popular, common treatments among many medical doctors who practice what is known as complementary medicine. Dr. Robert Gleser, former medical director at Pritikin Longevity Center and founder of Healthmark, a Colorado-based clinic advocating preventive medicine, routinely prescribes herbs for his patients who lack optimal energy balance. Recently adding a degree in Oriental medicine to his credentials, Gleser has put together a team consisting of medical doctors, herbal specialists, certified massage therapists, and acupuncturists. When evaluating the needs of his patients—which include many executives from the Rocky Mountain region—he says they "look at the energy balance of the body, checking to see where any imbalances are located, and how they should be treated." To help patients maintain optimal vitality, the team "correlates and develops a combined modality of treatment using whatever is appropriate, from medicine to herbs, or surgery to acupuncture."

In addition to common multivitamin preparations, phytochemicals or "super foods" extracted from fruits, vegetables, and other plants are being assessed for their ability to enhance health and well-being. The prescription of these exotic ingredients to support human vitality has spawned the emerging nutraceuticals industry (a nutraceutical is a food or a part of a food that offers medical and health benefits). Dr. Stephen DeFelice, founder of the Center for Innovation in Human Medicine, believes that ultimately one-half of the entire U.S. food supply will be fortified with nutraceuticals designed to optimize well-being. Nutritional products designer Brian Keating, President of the Seattle-based Sage Group, predicts that dietary supplements are especially valuable for businesspeople facing long hours and high pressure. "Scientifically formulated supplements made from herbs and various nutrients have been clinically proven to enhance oxygen flow to the brain, inhibit the effects of stress, and boost energy levels," Keating says. He cites ginseng, ginkgo biloba, and Saint-John's-wort as examples of clinically utilized natural ingredients that improve performance.

Road Warriors

Eating a healthy diet while on the road can be a challenge. Many times, you're in a hurry, you don't know any healthy restaurants, or you're eating out with clients. In some locations—such as smaller towns in the Midwest and South—people may raise an eye when you ask for yolkless eggs or unbuttered toast. (When recently in Wichita for a conference, a friend went to a restaurant and ordered his tuna "lightly seared." The waiter looked him up and down and said, "You're not from Wichita, are you?") Traveling internationally can sometimes make healthy eating habits even more problematic. Occasionally, eating well-balanced meals is just too inconvenient.

But with foresight and practice, you can eat well on the road and thereby enhance your ability to negotiate effectively and deliver great presentations. Remember, the goal is to help you stay in a composed, enthusiastic state so you can achieve maximum results from your meetings or sales calls. When you're on the road, you're on a mission; it's not the time to ignore healthy eating habits; it's the time to observe them more carefully.

EATING IN THE AIR

"How can you eat well with airline food?" numerous audience participants have asked me. While typical airline food makes it a challenge, maintaining healthy eating habits when traveling by plane is not overly difficult. With a twenty-four-hour notice, most airlines will substitute their traditional fare with a rather astounding array of meals, including vegetarian, seafood, kosher, Japanese, a fruit plate, or a low-fat, low-calorie, low-cholesterol meal. You, your travel agent, or your assistant should automatically choose one of these each time you fly. Usually, they're quite good—many times the people around me stare enviously at my fruit plate and resolve to special order on their next trip. If you don't call ahead, you always have the option of simply not eating the fatty items on the tray they put in front of you (reject it outright if you don't want to test your willpower), and get something healthier when you land.

Flying is dehydrating, so you should drink water and other nonalcoholic liquids on the plane to counteract this effect. If you want to drink alcoholic beverages, be aware that they have some potentially negative consequences. Depending on your system, alcohol can dehydrate you, destabilize your blood sugar levels, and combine with the altitude to produce unpleasant effects on your head later that night or the next morning.

Dinner is probably the toughest meal on the plane, because often you're tired and hungry after a long day of work. You're much better off buying a turkey sandwich in the airport and taking it on the plane than eating the typical dinner entrée. If you're relegated to the airline fare, try to eat the low-fat portion of the meal.

If you fly regularly and don't watch your food and beverage consumption, you can easily gain two to five pounds of fat per month. It's not worth it. Strategize.

LIFE IN THE DRIVE-THRU LANE

If you spend a lot of time driving to meetings or sales calls, you face a new set of problems, because by far the quickest and easiest way to eat is to stop at a convenience store or use the drive-thru of a fast-food restaurant. The typical fare at such establishments, however, makes you tired, slow-witted, and tense. I've talked with plenty of frequent drivers who start their day with doughnuts and coffee, follow that with a hamburger and fries at lunch, and stop for a candy bar and Coke in the afternoon. Whether you're making sales calls, visiting clients, or going to meetings, such a diet prepares you to make a less than impressive appearance.

You're always better off going into a restaurant and ordering low-fat foods like salads, turkey sandwiches, grilled chicken, or lean roast beef. For snacks while driving, take fruit, pretzels, bagels, or nonbuttered, preservative-free popcorn, and bottled water. Play upbeat jazz or your favorite music to stay energetic and alert. It's already tiring and nerve-fraying to handle traffic, directions, parking, and tight schedules—do yourself a favor and eat foods that will gear you up for the challenge rather than contribute to the tension.

Eat Like a Professional

To be a top performer in business, you simply have to have un-flagging levels of energy and optimism. Eating the right foods at the right times is one of the most practical, valuable strategies to boost your mind-set and success.

CATCHFIRE TIPS FOR EATING FOR PERFORMANCE

1. *Keep the right proportions.* Eat a diet consisting of approximately 65 percent carbohydrate, 15 percent protein, and 20 percent fat.
2. *Eat breakfast!* Make it low-fat and high in carbohydrates (oatmeal, cereal, fruit, bread, English muffins, or bagels).
3. *Graze, don't gorge.* Eat five or six smaller, lighter meals per day (three lighter meals plus two or three healthy snacks).
4. *Savor, don't scarf.* Eat mindfully for more pleasure and less overeating.

5. *Eat protein for mental alertness.* Make lunch high in protein to stay energized through the afternoon (chicken, turkey, fish, beans, lean beef).

6. *Eat carbohydrates to relax.* When eating later, eat lighter.

7. *Drink eight glasses of water per day.* Start with one at breakfast.

8. *Emphasize fresh fruit and vegetables.* In addition to eating fruit and vegetables with meals, have them at midmorning and midafternoon breaks.

9. *Avoid caffeine after noon.*

10. *Take vitamins.* Make use of moderate-dose vitamin and mineral supplements.

> *"When my creative energy flowed most freely,*
> *my muscular activity was always greatest . . .*
> *I might often have been seen dancing."*
> Friedrich Nietzsche

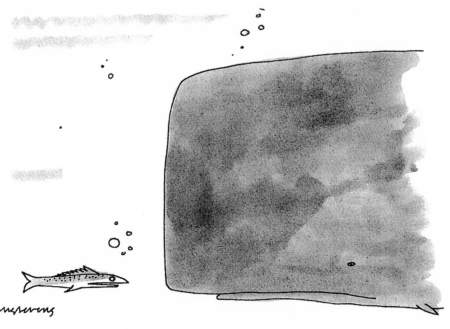

"Diet alone isn't enough—you also have to exercise."

STEP 3

Working Out to Work Better: Energy-Boosting, Stress-Busting Exercise

I am a great believer in the benefits of sensible, moderate exercise . . . from my own experience as one who hated exercise for much of his life and now does not feel right if a day goes by without some form of it.

—Andrew Weil, M.D.

"I t's hard for me to understand," says Jim Haymaker of Cargill, "how folks who don't work out on a regular basis are able to withstand the rigors of competition at firms, large or small, at today's pace—plus handle the huge tug of responsibilities between home, work, and community." Haymaker oversees the recruitment, training, and operations of Cargill's internal consulting department, a task that embroils him in endless meetings and interviews, sends him around the world to visit various business units, and requires numerous hours of reading, research, and analysis. To maintain high energy, sharp thinking, and a fresh perspective throughout his demanding schedule, he depends heavily on aerobic exercise.

Haymaker has integrated workouts into his lifestyle and usually looks forward to them. In the summer, he swims, jogs, bikes, and skates. During the Minnesota winter—which banishes the very thought of bikes and in-line skates—he goes to a health club to swim and work out. But as much as he likes the physical activity, he consciously uses exercise as a tool to prepare him to face the challenges of work. When traveling on business in Europe or Asia, for instance, Haymaker packs his jogging clothes and swimsuit, and gently forces his jet-lagged body and mind into a brief, reenergizing run or swim. "It would be hard for me to do this job without working out," Haymaker says. "It makes traveling internationally easier, but just in terms of the day-in-and-day-out grind, the amount of additional energy and perspective that it provides is hard to describe. Not to mention the fact of the long-term positive effects of being in shape and feeling more vibrant."

The Benefits of Exercise

An ever-growing mountain of research celebrates the virtues of exercise and warns against the risks of being sedentary. Regular aerobic activity, these studies show, reduces the incidence of heart disease and hypertension. It lowers cholesterol, enhances your immune system, and generally improves the functioning of almost every organ and system in your body. Not exercising, on the other hand, has the opposite effect. A sedentary lifestyle is associated with an increased rate of illness and disease of nearly every type, from the common cold to heart disease and stroke. One major study recently showed that chronic inactivity predisposes you to approximately the same risk of early death as smoking.

In addition to the well-publicized benefits to your physical condition, however, exercise has a more immediate and exciting advantage: it radically improves your ability to perform at work. Because of its impact on your productivity, exercise—Step 3 of the CatchFire program—plays a vitally important part in your business life. Studies on aerobic exercise show that it has a considerable, often dramatic effect on energy, tension, mood, and problem-solving abilities. In the long term, a sensible workout regimen reconditions your body in a way that enables it to produce energy more efficiently, respond to stress more productively, and think with greater clarity. Short term, 20 to 30 minutes of aerobic activity can create a change in biochemistry that launches you into a state of confidence and exhilaration. The overall effect of a good exercise program is to provide you with better fuel to think and a better engine to put it in—a powerful combination that ignites your ability to creatively solve problems, thrive under pressure, and perform at peak levels of effectiveness.

My research with businesspeople across the country not only reinforces these findings but also shows that many professionals share Jim Haymaker's zeal: physical activity is simply invaluable for consistently working at your best. In the Professional Workforce Survey, over two-thirds of the respondents reported that exercise contributes to their energy, attitude, and on-the-job performance. And many felt much more strongly about it: 53 percent said that exercise is "very important" to their energy level; almost half reported that working out plays a "very important" role in their overall attitude; and more than 40 percent of the professionals surveyed reported that exercise was a "very important" factor in their performance on the job. Comparing those who regularly work out to those who follow an inactive lifestyle was even more telling: people who regularly work out report significantly lower stress levels than those who rarely exercise, say they are more likely to attack problems with enthusiasm, and report themselves to be top performers in greater proportion to their sedentary counterparts. Finally, the well-exercised lot earns, on average, a higher household income than the inactive crowd.

As convincing as these numbers are, however, they pale beside the fervid endorsements of exercise offered in the interviews I conducted. In these conversations, frequent exercisers (which most of our interview subjects turned out to be) didn't just say that their workouts were important, they passionately swore by them. "I can't imagine *not* working out," said Paul Hoffman, the Vice President of Worldwide Sales at Documentum. "Exercise totally revives me" and "A great workout gives you an entirely new perspective" were sentiments that people invoked with frequency. Fredda McDonald,

President of Cadmus Marketing Services, a $33 million printing company in Atlanta, believes in exercise so strongly that she extended an open offer to her staff: "I'm supportive of you going to work out whenever you need to." The employees say working out at the nearby fitness facility is crucial to staying productive throughout their twelve- to fourteen-hour days; McDonald says she loves to see people return from a workout "all pumped up."

The consensus of the science, statistics, and testimony is that exercise is a devastatingly effective tool for erasing tension, injecting energy, and revitalizing a positive mood.

Making the Commitment

Despite the convincing research on exercise and the enthusiasm that devoted exercisers exhibit toward their habit, most people work out rarely or not at all. Government surveys, in fact, put the number of sedentary people at about 60 percent of the population (only 10 to 15 percent work out regularly). What's the problem? How can so many people know that exercise improves their bodies and minds, and yet not stick to a regular workout schedule? Most people say they don't have the time to work out. Many can't muster the energy to climb onto a stair machine after an exhausting day of work. Some think that aerobic exercise is boring. And a few still seem to believe that the fitness movement is a fad, clinging to the words of the comedian who said, "Whenever I feel the urge to exercise, I just lie down until the feeling goes away."

Starting an exercise program does require some time and effort. But it's not anywhere close to the pain-inflicting, time-consuming imposition that many nonexercisers make it out to be. In fact, the majority of people find that once they've begun a good exercise program, they begin to look forward to their workouts; sometimes their bike ride or aerobics class turns out to be one of the best parts of the day. Even if it doesn't become a major priority, an economical routine of three or four 30-minute sessions per week can produce substantial improvements in your energy level, confidence, and ability to work under pressure.

And not only can your workouts be relatively quick, if that's how you prefer them, but they also can be fun. For the majority of the exercise averse, the prospect of being lashed to a rowing machine and forced to repeatedly pull until they are sweating, red-faced, and exhausted calls forth the notion of torture far sooner than the notion of fun. But while you have to push yourself to reap the benefits of working out, pain has no place in a good exercise program. In fact, the opposite is true: enjoyment is a critical ingredient to any good workout program, and with solid background knowledge and a little imagination you can design an exercise program that keeps you interested and satisfied. Participating in activities you enjoy, varying your workouts, listening to music, using the opportunity to become more attuned to your body—by strategizing your attack, you can make exercise a vital and enjoyable part of your lifestyle.

By far the best approach is to make regular exercise a life-long commitment. Crash exercise programs, like crash diets, are doomed to fail. If you're out of shape, you can begin with some simple walking sessions and basic exercises that will boost your energy and mood right away, and pave the road to a more vigorous lifestyle. But making physical activity an integral part of every week of your life will increase your sense of vitality, enhance your self-image, and help you effectively handle the challenges of a chaotic business world.

Relearning to Move

Humankind was born to move. In the evolution of our species, the musculoskeletal system of humans—the one that orchestrates movement—developed millions of years before the brain and remains intricately connected to all other systems in the body. Because of the centrality of this system, movement, and especially vigorous movement, triggers a surge of biochemical changes that modifies not just your muscles and bones but also your immune system, mood, emotions, and thoughts.

Historically, our ancestors had plenty of physical activity in

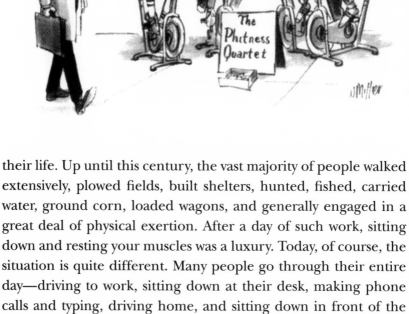

The Phitness Quartet

their life. Up until this century, the vast majority of people walked extensively, plowed fields, built shelters, hunted, fished, carried water, ground corn, loaded wagons, and generally engaged in a great deal of physical exertion. After a day of such work, sitting down and resting your muscles was a luxury. Today, of course, the situation is quite different. Many people go through their entire day—driving to work, sitting down at their desk, making phone calls and typing, driving home, and sitting down in front of the TV—without ever doing any moderately intensive physical activity. The routine can still be exhausting, but in terms of actively moving your body, most people follow a severely limited schedule.

So while the notion of working up a sweat as you pedal away on a stationary bike strikes some people, not unjustifiably, as highly curious, when viewed from an evolutionary perspective, the pattern of not using your body at all is the truly bewildering behavior. Compared to the lifestyles of our ancestors, our society unnaturally deprives itself of physical activity. This sedentary habit weakens the physical processes of the body and often leads to illness. And because of the interconnected nature of the muscular system, brain, and other processes of the body, being sedentary also depresses your mood, thinking, and your ability to work productively.

Fortunately, the antidote to this problem is clear. Initiating a well-designed exercise program creates a wave of positive changes in health and performance. Physically, you lose fat, build firm, lean muscle, increase your strength, and tone your body and skin. More to the point, aerobic exercise helps you build confidence, quell negative anxiety, work with a higher level of energy, and think with greater mental clarity and concentration. I consider it one of the best ways to enhance your personal performance in a challenging world of business. At the risk of sounding cliché—just do it.

Exercising for Energy

The vast array of physiological changes that occur during aerobic exercise provides a surge in energy level. Over the long run, regular aerobic activity reconditions your entire body to become a smooth, efficient, high-powered machine. In the short term—say, when you go for a run on your lunch hour—it unleashes a cascade of positive physiological effects, such as increased oxygen availability and a greater production of alertness biochemicals, that recharge your body and brain.

Another term for aerobic exercise is *systemic exercise*, or exercise that affects your entire system. This kind of exercise doesn't just alter the muscles used in the activity—your leg muscles as you jog, for instance—but significantly changes the heart, lungs, blood, bones, nervous system, brain, and most other organs throughout the body. Why do all these changes occur? Aerobic activity requires you to vigorously move your major muscle masses, breathe deeply but not so hard that you are out of breath, and maintain your exercise for at least 12 minutes. Activity that meets these three requirements makes major demands on your body, demands that initiate a whole series of changes. Among the most important: the liver and fat depositories release fuel, the heart pumps more blood, the lungs take in more oxygen, and the blood carries more oxygen and fuel to the muscles. The sum of these processes creates healthy changes in your energy level.

One of the most important long-term effects of these changes concerns your metabolism, or the rate at which you burn calories. Regularly riding your bike or using the stair machine stimulates the growth of the fat-burning enzymes inside your muscles, which means you burn more fat and increase the rate of your metabolism. A crucial aspect of the change is that this accelerated metabolic rate doesn't apply just during exercise; whether you are sitting at your desk or running in the park, the fit, metabolically advanced person burns more calories—and a greater percentage of fat calories—than the out-of-shape person. Since fat molecules store more energy than glucose (carbohydrate) molecules, burning a higher proportion of them releases more energy. Aerobic exercise, to put it another way, stokes your metabolic fire and creates a greater outpouring of light and heat.

The system seems almost unfair to those who are in poor physical condition. But the good news is that these critical fat-burning enzymes are what scientists call *inducible*—that is, you can induce them to grow or shrink. A good aerobic exercise program stimulates their growth and transforms your body into a more effective fuel burner. Resigning your health club membership and spending more time on the couch, on the other hand, causes them to contract and burn less fat as fuel. By some cruel quirk of nature, it's easier to slide back to a metabolically sluggish system than it is to induce an accelerated one. But as long as you maintain an ample degree of physical activity, you will lose fat, gain lean muscle, and permanently become a more efficient manufacturer of energy.

The immediate effects of aerobic exercise are equally exciting. As the veteran exerciser knows, aerobic activity exerts a rejuvenating effect on the body and mind. Even if you've worked a ten-hour day and feel exhausted, a good session at the gym can almost miraculously revive your spirits. This reaction might seem counterintuitive—that exerting yourself makes you feel more energetic. But the response illustrates an important principle about your energy level: you can't "save up" the feeling of being energetic by sitting still. Paradoxically, you have to expend energy to get more energy.

I want to emphasize this point for those who believe that exercise depletes your energy. It's a fallacy to think of energy as gas in a gas tank, which you can expend on various tasks—either working or playing with your kids or exercising—until it runs out. Of course, you burn calories when you go for a swim or a walk. But unless you overexert yourself, the systemic changes that accompany this calorie-burning activity don't deplete your energy, but instead stimulate a higher level of vitality, alertness, and enthusiasm.

Marty Paradise, Microsoft's Regional Manager in Atlanta, finds that his workouts have just such a regenerative effect. "Sometimes you think, 'I'm going to be a lot more tired if I get up earlier to work out in the morning,' " he says. "But I find I'm a lot more energetic, even if I have to get up early to go work out. It works that way." Paradise wasn't always in great shape—in fact, for many years, he didn't follow an exercise program at all. But once he started, he pursued his physical conditioning with rare enthusiasm and dedication. When he was working as District Manager at Microsoft's Phoenix office, Paradise started a routine where he and his associates would meet most days at 5:30 A.M. to climb nearby Camelback Mountain. And while Paradise has had to replace hiking in the mountains with a stair machine in Atlanta, he says his morning workouts put him in a high-energy state for the rest of the day: "It loosens me up, it makes me feel better about myself, and I have more energy to perform at work."

John Saeman also depends on his workouts to provide a rejuvenating energy boost. Saeman, the former CEO of the cable company Daniels & Associates, now owns Medallion Enterprises, L.L.C. At age 60, he undertakes a formidable schedule of work and travel—and a vigorous exercise program. Aside from just exercising when he feels like he has the energy, Saeman uses workouts for their transforming effect. "When I feel crabby, I just don't want to work out. But that's when I need to most, because it pulls me through," Saeman says. "If I can get on the machine and work out for forty minutes, it's just like taking an upper. I feel great afterward." Though his typical workout routine—with stretching, forty minutes of aerobics on a treadmill, and abdomen crunches—

runs about an hour and ten minutes, Saeman says he can revitalize his energy level with an abbreviated version: "If I get home and I know we have to go out that night, I'll get on the treadmill machine—even if it's only for ten or twenty minutes—and go hard, take a shower, and feel totally refreshed."

While scientists don't know exactly what goes on in the body and brain to produce the energy surge that Saeman and Paradise describe, they know about a few of the key players. Elevated levels of blood oxygen, for example, contribute to the infusion of vitality. And a temporary influx of the neurochemicals endorphin, dopamine, serotonin, and norepinephrine play a role as well. Whatever the exact molecular modulations, the sum of these changes in chemistry creates a feeling of exuberance that endures long after you finish your workout.

Elevating Your Mood

In addition to its impact on energy, aerobic exercise can bring about a decisive transformation in attitude. Over the long term, regular aerobic activity has the remarkable effect of fine-tuning the body's response to stress, so you react to challenges with an appropriate amount of energy and attention. More immediately, it acts as a potent stimulant to your mood, creating a change in biochemistry that leaves you feeling calm, confident, and joyful. In fact, because of numerous studies that demonstrate a positive effect, many psychologists prescribe exercise to depressed patients as part of their therapy.

Physically fit people respond to high-pressure situations more effectively. Exercise activates the release of the "stress" neurochemicals epinephrine and norepinephrine into the bloodstream, which signals the body to breathe faster, pump more blood, and release more fat and glucose to use as fuel. But as you begin to exercise regularly and get into good physical condition, you train your body to reduce the traffic of stress neurochemicals—both resting levels of the chemicals and the amount your body releases while working out. You still produce the needed increases in oxygen and fuel when you play tennis or go for a bike ride. But getting in shape enables your system to acquire a greater subtlety in its response to the demands of exercise, so it produces only the changes in chemistry and physiology that are necessary.

What's exciting is that aerobic exercise serves not only as physical training but as emotional training as well. That is, just as several weeks of jogging enables you to handle a three-mile run with less huffing and puffing, pain, and struggle, it also helps you deal with the pressure of a tight deadline or a difficult customer with less tension, frustration, and irritability. A feeling that you can cope predominates; you don't get nervous or frustrated. Because aerobically fit people have lower resting levels of stress neurochemicals, they bypass feelings of anxiety and address their problems with greater flexibility and poise.

To be clear, exercise doesn't depress your body's stress arousal mechanism, which in many ways serves necessary and beneficial purposes. Instead, aerobic activity refines it. Once you've been exercising regularly for some time, you possess a greater physiological and psychological ability to stay composed when you encounter everyday emotional stress, such as a heavy workload or an uncooperative teammate. On the other hand, you respond with a heightened degree of alertness when you're facing a new situation that demands a higher level of attention. Overall, regular aerobic exercise doesn't just strengthen and tone your body; it shapes up your mood and emotions in a way that helps you deal with stressful situations more productively.

In addition to equipping your body with an improved pressure-handling capacity, a good session of aerobic activity produces an immediate burst of positive emotion. While the reason you experience mild euphoria or "runner's high" after exercise isn't known precisely, the increased presence of the neurochemical endorphin plays a major role. Heightened endorphin levels in the brain stimulate a sense of calmness and well-being. Even if you're frustrated, mentally exhausted, and forlorn, dragging yourself into the gym for an endorphin-elevating workout enables you to emerge confident, joyful, and profoundly refreshed. Triggering this change in attitude, especially if you're in the midst of stressful changes or nerve-racking deals, can have an enormous impact on your performance.

Halyna Doherty of Mutual Life of Canada, for instance, strategically employs her workouts to help her remain confident and upbeat through some of her toughest assignments as Marketing Services Officer. "If I am feeling challenged and I have half an hour or forty-five minutes, I go down to our fitness center and I work out," Doherty says. "I feel that if I sit at my desk and stare, or go grab a coffee, that's not going to help. I need to get away and get my blood flowing." Recently, during an intense series of budget and salary-change discussions she conducted, the workouts enabled her to maintain her poise and productivity. "When I come back from a workout, I have a different perspective," Doherty says. "I feel better, it clears my mind, and I think a lot clearer. It really works."

Jump-Starting Your Thinking

Exercise also helps you think with greater acuity and creativity. During aerobic exercise, you dramatically increase your oxygen uptake, as well as the production of the red corpuscles that carry oxygen to the brain. This influx of blood oxygen enhances the functioning of every organ in your body. And because a hefty 25 percent of your blood is in the brain at any one time, your thinking power receives a forceful boost (a fact that many experiments involving exercise and mental performance have demonstrated). In addition to the increased oxygen, the right side of the brain—the one specializing in recognizing new patterns and pictures—becomes more active when you exercise. Combined, these two changes pack a powerful creative problem-solving punch.

I've always liked the old Hewlett-Packard television commercial that dramatizes this effect. In the commercial, an executive at her desk is unable to come up with a solution to her marketing problem. Throwing down her pen in disgust, she bolts from the office to take a swim. We catch her toweling off by the pool; she stops,

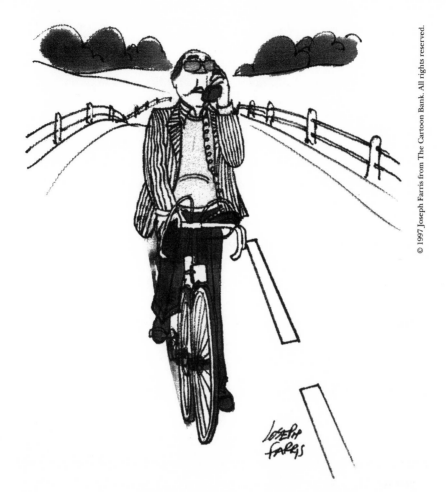

rushes to a conveniently placed phone, dials a number, and says, "What if . . ."

Marie Amoruso, who was Director of Planning when I worked with her at Apple Computer and is now Vice President of Marketing for Taligent, could have been the prototype for this commercial. In the midst of a hectic atmosphere, Amoruso uses exercise to relieve feelings of anxiety and to engender a productive mental state. As she says, "I can't be in a frenzied mode—there has to be calm around me." For Amoruso, an occasional exercise break is so important that she will rearrange her schedule to make time for a workout. "If I really get stressed out, I will cancel an appointment and go for a run," Amoruso says. "Instead of thinking, 'If I take an hour now, it's going to take me longer to get home,' I take the responsibility and give myself permission to take that hour off, because I know it will help my thinking and decision making."

Pat O'Donnell, the CEO of Aspen Skiing Company, has come to count on his workouts to provide him with new ideas. Every morning at 4 A.M., he exercises for an hour and a half, doing a combination of aerobics, weight lifting, and stretching. While he realizes the benefits of working out to his health and energy level, O'Donnell says the time has become a crucial period of idea germination: "That's when I do a lot of my thinking. As a matter of fact, it's almost ridiculous now because I take a little notepad from station to station." But unquestionably, O'Donnell says, it works. "I usually walk out with six or seven thoughts on a piece of paper."

Designing an Optimal Exercise Program

Most physical activity—whether it's running, weight lifting, playing tennis, or doing yoga—confers at least some benefit to both your physical health and your mood. But often, the activities people engage in don't maximize energy, reduce tension, and enhance performance. Exercising to achieve these goals requires an emphasis on aerobic activity, and a constant bias toward keeping your activities balanced and fun. By modifying your aerobic activity with techniques such as cross training and interval training, and incorporating activities such as weight-bearing and flexibility exercises, you can substantially improve the effectiveness of your workouts. And as a result, you can energize your performance at work.

Setting an exercise program—or revamping an anemic one— that reaps such benefits demands that you take a strategic approach. One of the primary elements of this strategy is to make exercise a lifelong commitment. Rather than adopting a "take no prisoners" mentality and trying to beat better health into your body by lifting immense barbells and running ten miles a day (a program that would probably collapse inside of two weeks), you have to begin with the intention of incorporating exercise into every week of your life. With that in mind, start slowly, learn new information, experiment with different exercises, and gradually progress to longer periods of exercise and higher levels of intensity. As the Zen master told the snail, "Oh, snail, climb Mount Fuji, but slowly, slowly." (This advice is critical if you're greatly out of shape.)

Doing exercise you enjoy is another vital element of your exercise strategy. If you don't make your workouts fun—varying your exercises, enlisting friends and family in your activities, listening to music, playing sports, exercising in pleasant indoor or outdoor settings—you will very likely quit. Beyond increasing the longevity of your program, having fun actually improves the physical benefits you get from your workout. Studies conducted by Dr. Lee Berk and Dr. Stanley Tan at Loma Linda University show that people who enjoy their exercise (or at least approach it with a positive attitude) produce more healthy biochemical changes, lose more fat, and more significantly enhance their lung capacity than those who find the experience to be miserable. To some extent, you learn to like exercise as you learn to like tennis or skiing—by doing it and getting better at it. But making your physical activity enjoyable isn't just helpful, it's essential to the physiological benefits of your workout.

The best way to begin an exercise program is to get a fitness physical, which can be performed by your doctor, a health club, or, if you're lucky, your company's wellness center. Dr. Robert Gleser of Healthmark describes an ideal fitness physical as one that tests the following: cholesterol, EKG stress test, VO_2 max, fat/lean body composition, blood pressure, and resting heart rate (which are various tests of the proficiency of your heart, lungs, and blood). This examination allows you to assess any potential risk factors in your exercise program, and set realistic goals for health and performance. Moreover, a fitness physical significantly raises your awareness of your body's fitness level, and acts like a rite of passage from a sedentary life to a new life of health and energy. It isn't absolutely necessary, but at the very least, I think you'll find the results interesting and motivating.

THE ELEMENTS OF AN IDEAL WORKOUT SCHEDULE

While a wide variety of physical activity can improve your health, the following guidelines produce the physical and mental transformations that enable you to work at your best:

1. Aerobic Exercise
   - Minimum three times per week, 20 minutes each time
   - Preferably four or five times a week
   - Cross training—alternate the type of exercise
   - Interval training—alternate the intensity of exercise
2. Weight-bearing Exercise
   - Minimum of two times per week, 10 minutes each time
   - Preferably four or five times per week
   - Include abdomen crunches (mini sit-ups)
3. Flexibility Exercise
   - Minimum of two times per week, 10 minutes per time
   - Preferably four or five times per week

AEROBIC EXERCISE

The heart of an energy-boosting, mood-enhancing exercise program is aerobic exercise. Aerobic exercise, to reiterate, is activity that meets three conditions: it uses the major muscles, specifically the thighs or buttocks; it causes you to breathe deeply but not run out of breath; and it is sustained for a period of at least 12 minutes—although incorporating a 20- to 30-minute session into your workout is preferable. Examples of aerobic exercise include running, brisk walking, biking, swimming, and using exercise machines such as stair machines, treadmills, and stationary bikes. Some sports are aerobic and some are not. While it depends on the intensity with which you play, full-court basketball and soccer are usually aerobic; softball, tennis, volleyball, and golf—though all have physiological merit—are not.

All aerobic exercise should commence with a 5-minute warm-up period and end with a 5-minute cool-down session. (The warm-up and cool-down consists of simply doing slowly whatever you're going to do for your aerobic exercise—if your activity is jogging, start by jogging slowly in order to warm up your muscles.)

FREQUENCY OF AEROBIC EXERCISE

Research recommends exercising a minimum of three times a week. Working out three times per week provides well-documented benefits for your heart, lungs, bones, and overall health. I encourage you, if you've reached a comfortable level of fitness, to aim higher. I try to do something active every day. That doesn't mean I actually run or go to the gym, but if I don't get a formal workout in—which I do about five times per week—then I at least go for a walk after dinner or do some light calisthenics at home (or in my hotel room).

If you're committed to more energy, greater confidence, and better performance, shoot for four to five workouts per week. Don't push yourself too hard, or develop an obsession with exercise, or feel guilty if you miss a couple of workouts. But if you follow a sensible exercise program, each workout will recharge your mood and contribute to your sense of self-assurance. Especially if you're facing tough demands every day at the office, exercising is an ideal way to keep you in the energy zone throughout your challenges.

EXERCISE INTENSITY

How hard should you work out? The typical answer is that you should exercise at 65 to 80 percent of your maximum heart rate. In this zone—your "target heart rate"—your muscles are moving, you're breathing deeply, your blood is delivering ample amounts of oxygen, and you're burning fat as your major fuel source.

The formula for determining your target heart rate is to

subtract your age from 220—which is your "maximum heart rate"—and then multiply that number by 65 to 80 percent. The target heart rate for a 40-year-old, then, would be between 117 (180 × .65) and 144 (180 × .80).

The much more practical way to keep track of your exercise intensity is this: exercise at a level where you are breathing deeply but comfortably enough so you can hold a conversation.

If you don't exercise hard enough to get your heart rate up, you won't produce the changes in your body and brain that recharge your energy level and mood. Exercising harder than your target heart rate, however—to the point where you can't speak a full sentence without gasping—can also diminish the effectiveness of your workout. While elite athletes regularly train with their heart rates at levels higher than 80 percent of their maximum, the purpose is to help them get their bodies in a superior physical condition to perform a specialized sport or activity.

For the person exercising to improve energy and performance, working out at such elevated levels has two major drawbacks. First, it causes you to burn more glucose than fat as an energy source, which can detract from fat loss and from the conditioning of your body. And second, it can leave you feeling tired rather than exhilarated after your workout. For most people, pushing yourself to the limit is unwise and ineffective.

CROSS TRAINING

Cross training is a technique that you can add to your aerobic fitness routine that drives up the effectiveness of your workouts. Cross training consists, very simply, of alternating the aerobic activities you do. Instead of using a stair machine four days a week, for example, use it for two or three, and alternate it with a day or two of biking. Instead of running five times a week, run for two, swim for two, and go for a hike one day. Which activities you substitute doesn't matter—as long as they are aerobic.

Cross training provides a more effective workout because the body perceives different forms of exercise as more demanding— even if it doesn't *seem* more demanding—and responds with greater internal exertion. As a result of this exertion, you use more fat as your fuel source and become a more efficient calorie burner and energy producer.

INTERVAL TRAINING

Interval training is another technique that increases the effectiveness of your exercise. Interval training simply means varying the intensity at which you exercise. Many elite athletes use heart rate monitors to help them with their interval training; they modulate the intensity of their workout according to specific guidelines in an effort to boost their endurance and performance. While you don't need to go to such lengths, you can use interval training to create significant gains in your fitness and energy levels.

Interval training works for people at all points of the fitness spectrum. Even if you're starting an exercise program for the first time, and you're beginning with, say, three 30-minute walks per week, you can still get the benefits of interval training. Walk briskly for 5 minutes or so and then go just a bit faster—until you're almost out of breath. Then slow back down to your original pace, and repeat the process in another 5 minutes. When I run outside, I slowly jog, then pick up the pace to a run for maybe a minute, and then return to a slow jog—alternating for the entire 30 minutes or so that I exercise.

If you use aerobic machines, you can either choose the interval programs already programmed into the machine or manually adjust your speed to get the interval training benefits. Most people find that in addition to being more efficient exercise, adding interval training makes the activity more fun—or, if you have a hard time calling that fun, it's at least more interesting.

WEIGHT-BEARING EXERCISE

Weight-bearing exercise, also called *resistance training*, doesn't necessarily involve huge weights and isn't necessarily for building big muscles—I'm not recommending them for that purpose. In addition to toning your muscles and strengthening your bones, occasional weight-bearing exercises, when combined with aerobic exercise, drive up your fitness level. Weight-bearing exercise makes demands on the muscle that change its chemistry, making your body a more efficient energy producer.

There are a number of ways to do weight-bearing exercise. If you use weights, be sure to work with a knowledgeable fitness instructor to devise a routine of safe, effective lifting techniques. But you don't actually need to use weights to do weight-bearing exercise. Push-ups, abdomen crunches, "weightless" leg squats, and other calisthenics are weight-bearing activities—you're just bearing your own weight. (These exercises, by the way, are ideal for beginners, or for those who don't want to work out with weights.)

I recommend doing at least 10 minutes of weight-bearing exercises at least twice each week—I like to do at least one muscle group each time I go to the gym. The one exercise I urge you to do is abdomen crunches. These mini sit-ups strengthen your stomach muscles and back, and thereby promote good posture and less back pain. Try to incorporate two or three sets of ab crunches into each workout.

FLEXIBILITY EXERCISES (STRETCHING)

Without going through the numerous stretching routines and yoga exercises (there are plenty of good, amply illustrated books on these subjects), I want to emphasize that stretching not only protects you from injury but also is an excellent way to reduce muscle tension and promote physical and mental relaxation.

Try to do at least 10 minutes of stretching with each workout. But don't stretch cold muscles—stretch after a light warm-up (such as running in place) or after your workout.

TIME

There isn't any specific duration that your workouts should run. In fact, it varies widely depending on your activities and the intensity at which you perform them (you have to walk for about 45 minutes to get the equivalent workout of running 20 minutes). The minimum amount of time you need to spend doing aerobic exercise in order to produce performance-enhancing physiological effects is 12 minutes at an aerobic level of intensity. But if you've reached a moderate level of fitness, I encourage you to aim for at least 20 minutes of aerobic activity per workout. And if you're in great physical condition, I recommend that, at least occasionally, you go for half an hour or more.

In addition to 20 minutes of aerobic exercise, try to do approximately 10 minutes of weight-bearing exercise and 10 minutes of flexibility exercise per workout. This routine will drive up your fitness level and produce changes in your muscular system that will contribute greatly to your vitality, tension control, and performance.

As a rough guideline, then, you can do a rejuvenating, well-balanced workout in about 40 minutes—20 minutes of aerobics, 10 minutes of weight-bearing exercise, and 10 minutes of flexibility exercises. But again, the right amount of time depends heavily on your exercise goals and your schedule. If you are lifting weights in an attempt to build muscle, then you will obviously spend more time on that activity. If your schedule won't permit a 40-minute workout today, go for 20 minutes.

TIME OF DAY

In terms of the physiological benefits, it doesn't matter what time of day you exercise. The best time is when you can do it consistently and conveniently, and get the maximum advantage from its revitalizing effects.

Many people who have exceptionally busy schedules find that the only time they can regularly work out is in the morning. Aside from the fact that few duties will sidetrack you at 5:30 A.M., a morning run or workout puts you in a positive energy state for the entire day.

Executives I've talked to who exercise at some point during the workday almost unanimously report an immediate upsurge in energy and confidence. Unfortunately, this practice is inconvenient for many people: they lack the time or the fitness center, or the prospect of sweating before their three o'clock appointment

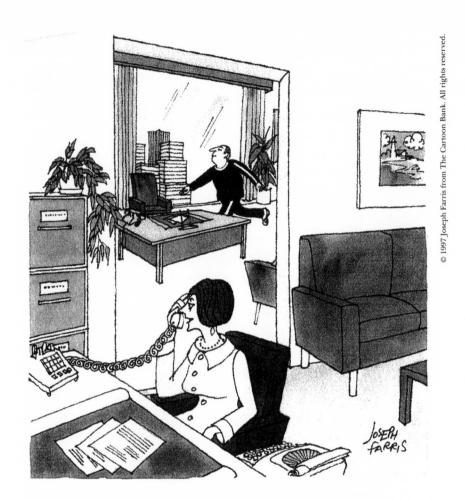

"Mr. Becerley can't talk to you now. He's jogging."

doesn't appeal to them. Try to at least reserve daily exercise as an option, so if the circumstances warrant and the time allows, you can bolt to the fitness center and dissolve your frustration on the treadmill. If a workout—or a short workout—is out of the question, incorporate a brisk 10- to 15-minute walk into your schedule when you need a shot of energy, optimism, and mental clarity.

Exercising after work has its benefits as well. At the end of a long day, a workout can reset your mood so you're ready for a great evening with your spouse and family. I find it a perfect activity with which to make the transition from office to home. One caveat, however: some people find that working out later in the day interferes with their sleep. Pay attention to your exercise and sleep patterns, and if you find that evening workouts keep you awake at night, work out earlier in the day. (But don't *stop* exercising. As we'll see in the next chapter, aerobic exercise, in general, helps you sleep better.)

HEALTH CLUBS VS. OUTDOORS

Another consideration in exercise strategy is whether to do it outdoors or indoors. Of course, it's not an "either/or" option; in fact, I urge you to choose both. While I play tennis, run, and bike, I also joined Kinetic Fitness Studio—a small workout facility in Denver—so I could vary my exercise and stay warm in the winter. Obviously, there is cost involved in joining a health club, and if you're an avid runner, biker, hiker, or in-line skater, then you don't really need to go inside for your aerobic activity. But the flexibility and variety of a health club makes it great to have as an option, especially if you live in an area where outdoor exercise isn't practical.

Finding a fitness center that has knowledgeable people and a pleasant atmosphere makes a big difference in terms of your motivation and the quality of your workouts. I chose mine because of the enthusiasm of Gene Cisneros, the owner and director of the facility, and the other enjoyable people who work out there. Cisneros keeps the exercise intense and fun, continually brings in new exercise machines, holds various exercise competitions, and plays good music.

Outdoor exercise has many benefits as well. Since most people spend most of their time indoors, a brisk walk, jog, or bike ride gives you a chance to enjoy sunshine and fresh air. In addition, running, biking, and playing sports require you to constantly balance your body as you run or play—something that exercise machines don't require of you. The act of balancing yourself and coordinating your muscles for a soccer kick or basketball shot actually takes a great deal of energy, and helps to drive up your fitness level. The drawbacks of outdoor exercise are bad weather, no weight-lifting facilities, and for some major metropolitan city-dwellers, no fresh air.

Before I discuss a number of different exercises, let me offer a final word of encouragement. Whether it's early morning, noon, or evening, sometimes you feel worn out before your designated workout time, and the last thing you want to do is climb on a bicycle or stair machine. At times like these, you have to concentrate on the surge of energy and elation you'll feel walking out of the gym after your workout. I think back to times when a workout has revived me, and I consider the fact that every time I've exercised, no matter how I felt beforehand, I ended up feeling refreshed when I finished. Start slowly, if you need to. In less than 10 minutes into the exercise, the biochemical changes kick in and before you know it, you start to feel great. Whether you're headed home or back to the office, you'll feel revitalized.

Which Exercises Are Best?

With the above parameters in mind, the following section discusses the relative merits and drawbacks of specific exercises.

WALKING

Walking is the easiest exercise and, along with swimming, the least likely to cause injury. To get aerobic benefits, however, you have to walk fast enough and far enough—generally, you should aim for 45 minutes at a brisk pace.

Walking is the best way to start your exercise program if you're in poor physical condition. Start by walking one or two miles at a slow pace, and gradually increase your distance and speed as you begin to feel more comfortable. As you get in better shape, incorporate interval training into your walks—intermittently pick up the pace until you're almost out of breath, and then slow down to your regular walking speed.

RUNNING/JOGGING

Running is an excellent exercise because of its intensity, which helps you quickly boost your fitness level. A 20- to 30-minute run makes an excellent, efficient workout. Its main drawback is that it can cause soreness or injury to your knees and back.

There's something that running does for me that nothing else quite matches. Because running on pavement more often than a couple of times a week causes soreness in my knees, I run outside six times a month at the most. In addition, I run on a treadmill a few times a week. Unfailingly, I have a more optimistic view of life after the exercise.

If you like to run but you're wary of the potential damage to your knees, there are machines that simulate running but exclude the jarring effect of pounding the pavement. These machines utilize full arm and leg motion, and they're comparatively easy to use, so they're good for beginners.

BICYCLING

Bicycling on a paved road falls somewhere in between walking and running in terms of intensity—depending, of course, on how fast you ride. While it's very easy on the joints of your legs (people coming back from knee surgery usually start back into exercise by biking), it gives your thighs and calves a great workout. Try to ride for at least 30 minutes at a brisk pace.

AEROBICS CLASSES

For a long time, because my schedule allowed it, aerobics classes were my major form of exercise. The camaraderie and group energy of aerobics classes add immeasurably to the interest and exhilaration, taking the focus off the fact that you are exerting yourself. If you get a good instructor who plays the right music, your workout will sometimes be the highlight of your day.

There is an endless variety of aerobics classes, from step classes to low-impact aerobics. Good classes are conducted so you can go at your own pace. While you may be reluctant to sign up if you're a beginner, the group enthusiasm of an aerobics class makes it a great way to start an exercise program.

SWIMMING

Swimming is a great complete-body exercise. It presents very low risk of injury, and can be a terrific way to work out for those who have injuries that are aggravated by other forms of exercise.

Swimming, however, does not stimulate fat loss. For reasons not totally understood, your muscles don't burn much fat as fuel when you're in water. If you're an avid swimmer, try to cross train with running or other "land" exercises to optimize the benefits of your exercise program.

OTHER SPORTS

Playing sports is a great way to keep your exercise fun. As long as you don't take them too seriously, they can provide a great source of healthy competition. And because coordinating your movements requires a kind of effort not necessary on exercise machines, they make a terrific cross-training activity to complement indoor aerobic exercise.

But as I mentioned, not all sports qualify as aerobic activity. While less active sports afford a moderate degree of physiological benefit, they don't produce the changes in your body and brain that lead to improvements in energy and performance.

To know whether a sport you play is aerobic, ask the following questions: Do you continuously move your major muscle masses (do you continuously run around)? Are you continually breathing deeply but not out of breath? Do you sustain a moderate degree of intensity for at least 20 minutes? Based on these guidelines, basketball, soccer, hockey, racquetball, water polo, and lacrosse are usually aerobic. Tennis, football, and volleyball aren't usually aerobic. And softball, baseball, and golf—unless you run in place the entire time—don't qualify as aerobic activities.

EXERCISE MACHINES

Stair-climbing machines are great for your legs and buttocks—and seem particularly effective at making you sweat. Select an interval training program if the machine you use has one in its computer; if not, manually vary your speed to make your exercise more effective.

Cross-country skiing and its more convenient counterpart, the cross-country ski machine, require the use of arms, legs, and shoulders, and thus very effectively promote fitness. (As a general rule, the more muscles you use, the more fat-burning enzymes you build, and the greater your level of fitness.)

Like cross-country ski machines, rowing machines are effective because they require several muscle groups—the legs, arms, and back. But take the time to learn the proper rowing technique so you don't cause soreness or injury to your back.

Stationary bikes give the legs a great workout. Many newer models include an arm-exercising apparatus as well, which gives you a great total body workout. I have a black and silver Schwinn Air-Dyne in my home (appropriately situated next to a painting by Miró, framed in black). I have a rule that I ride the bike for the first quarter of any sporting event that I'm watching on TV. And I usually spend one to two hours a week on it, in addition to my normal workouts.

Road Warriors— Traveling Is No Excuse

William Merriken, Senior Vice President at Polo Retail Corporation, firmly believes that working out enables people to perform with more enthusiasm and focus. "I do half an hour of aerobic exercise and half an hour of weights. I exercise six days a week in the morning, which is the only way I can control my time." Merriken's primary responsibility is to orchestrate an aggressive campaign to open Polo stores across the country. The campaign will raise the total number of their stores from twenty-two to well over thirty in the next couple of years, and it requires Merriken to spend a great deal of time on the road.

I asked Merriken if he kept up his exercise and healthy eating when he traveled, or, like most people, he suspended his health routine when he was on the road. "People use traveling as an excuse to allow themselves to 'tank,' " Merriken said. But he doesn't buy it. "Forget it. There's no excuse. I can go almost anywhere and eat and exercise the right way."

Travel often presents a great challenge to your exercise program.

As one who has logged over a million miles in the last eight years while following a fairly demanding workout schedule, I've encountered all the inconveniences that plague the nomadic exerciser. Jet lag, a busy schedule, and subpar workout facilities conspire to discourage you from working out. But usually your performance in different cities and countries is crucial—presumably important enough to pay for an airplane ticket and a hotel room. Whether you're meeting with people from a different branch of your company, making a sales presentation, or providing personal customer service, you have to think on your feet and win people over. This is the time, in other words, when exercise is most beneficial.

With greater awareness, preparation, and flexibility, you can devise an on-the-road workout routine that will maintain your exercise program and enhance your energy and alertness. If I get in the night before I do a presentation, I steadfastly ignore the bar—which calls to the exhausted traveler like the sirens to the weary Odysseus—go to my room, change into my workout clothes, and coax myself into a brief run, walk, swim, or workout. In short order, renewed confidence and enthusiasm supplant any jet lag or concern, and I'm primed to fully participate in whatever meetings or dinners are on the agenda.

In general, the best way to fit exercise into your work schedule when you're on the road is to do it in the morning. Use the hotel's workout facilities or go for a run (or a walk) and take a look around your new environment. Obviously, these activities will work equally well in the evening; but often, another engagement will interfere with this time. At the very least, do some calisthenics and stretching in your hotel room. A good 10- or 20-minute session of push-ups, abdomen crunches, and stretching will provide a noticeable boost in your energy and mood.

Reversing "Terminal Illness"

A well-executed workout is one of the best antidotes to the ills of the modern workplace—sitting at a desk all day long in front of a terminal, pushing to solve problems and meet deadlines. In the long run, a good exercise program is tremendously beneficial to maintaining the vigor of your body and brain. In the short run, exercise gives you a shot of confidence, clears out the cobwebs of your mind, and engenders a revitalized, more optimistic perspective of the world.

CATCHFIRE TIPS FOR WORKING OUT

1. *Start your exercise program with a strategy session.* Get a fitness physical. Outline your goals, and the what, when, where, and how of your strategy to achieve them.
2. *If you're a beginner, start by walking.* Go outside if possible, or use a treadmill indoors.
3. *Exercise regularly.* Try to do at least three or four workouts a week that include at least 20 minutes of aerobic exercise.
4. *Cross-train.* Do two or more different types of aerobic exercise.
5. *Use interval training.* Vary the intensity of your exercise.
6. *Raise your heart rate.* Exercise so you're breathing deeply and comfortably, but not out of breath.
7. *Add variety.* Incorporate weight-bearing and stretching exercises.
8. *Use whatever time you have.* If you can spare only 15 minutes, exercise for 15 minutes.
9. *Exercise to revitalize.* If you're feeling too tired but you're not exhausted or ill, force yourself to the gym, start slowly, and feel the reenergizing effect.
10. *Make it fun.* Vary your activities, listen to music, play sports, go hiking, involve your family and friends.

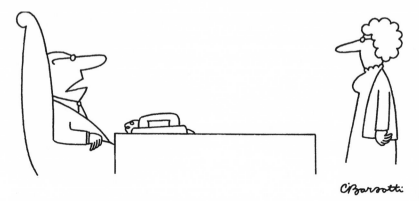

"*Miss Haskell, it's come to my attention that I've never had an original thought in my life, so I'm taking tomorrow off.*"

STEP 4
Breaking Up Stress and Fatigue: Breaks, Relaxation, and Sleep

We live in very difficult times, when man is faced with anxieties caused by rapid change. . . . We must find within our own bodies a physiologic means of dealing with the demands of twentieth-century life.

— Dr. Herbert Benson

The ancient Greek historian Herodotus recorded a brief account of the habits of a great Egyptian king named Amasis. King Amasis had a daily routine of working assiduously from dawn until noon, at which time he would abruptly quit whatever meetings or court proceedings were going on and retire for an afternoon of leisure. He and his cohorts told stories, traded witticisms, played games, and partook of the free-flowing barley brew. Decorum wasn't a foremost priority in the afternoon activities: according to Herodotus, some of the good king's jokes were "not seemly."

One day, the advisers to King Amasis informed him that some people looked unfavorably upon his routine. These folks, the advisers related, thought a king ought to act more dignified, in a manner that befitted his royal stature. The king listened politely as his advisers pleaded their case, and then replied, "When an archer goes into battle, he strings his bow until it is taut. When the shooting is over, he unstrings it again. If he didn't unstring it, it would lose its snap, and it would be no good to him when he needed it."

Herodotus says no more about Amasis, but he reports that his reign was the most prosperous in the history of Egypt.

Optimizing Your Performance by Doing Nothing

Rest and relaxation have fallen on hard times. As "doing more with less" has become the theme—or at least a prominent motif—in business, uninterrupted activity seems to have become the standard (certainly a different situation than if old King Amasis were at the helm). Stiffer competition, greater complexity, and shorter turnaround times have created an atmosphere that is sometimes thrilling, sometimes straining, but always really damn busy.

And it's not just that the pace of work at the office has intensified; work has expanded like a rising tide to fill more and more hours of the day. Staying at the office until well past 5 o'clock isn't unusual. Taking work home has become a popular habit. Saturdays and Sundays, for some people, represent a chance to catch up on what they didn't get done in the preceding five days, or an opportunity to prepare for the upcoming round of assignments. As a brief example of what seems a common schedule, witness the daily routine of Glenda Haines (a manager in the marketing department at Public Service Company of Colorado): "I get up a little before five A.M. to work out, I get to the office at eight, and I often work until eight or nine o'clock at night." To accommodate this surge of industriousness, a large segment of the population has slashed much of their time for breaks, relaxation, sleep, vacations, and interests outside of business.

Hard work can be exhilarating and rewarding. Undertaken with the proper enthusiasm, humor, and attention to health, difficult challenges can strengthen and enrich you. The problem is that many people aren't smart about the way they work. They push themselves into prolonged periods of exertion without adequate intervals of rest and relaxation. Some bulldoze their way through long days with a scant 5 minutes for lunch. Many chronically deny themselves sufficient hours of sleep. And some push themselves for months on end without taking a vacation—or even, in the extreme case, a solid work-free weekend. This relentlessly hard-driving approach, however, often proves self-defeating; for most people, it causes a decline in enthusiasm and concentration that diminishes their effectiveness.

In case it's not obvious, the body and mind don't function well when you rigorously run them without rest through an extensive obstacle course of phone calls, meetings, paperwork, negotiations, and presentations. Scientists call the extreme form of this intense, unremitting exertion "chronic stress." And as a wealth of research indicates, it undermines both your health and your performance. Physically, chronic stress can lead to a greater incidence of illness and burnout. Mentally and emotionally, it makes you tense, tired, scattered, and flat. King Amasis had it exactly right: if you don't unstring your bow, you quickly lose your snap.

Step 4 of the CatchFire program—implementing a new schedule of rest and relaxation—helps you reduce tension and illness, and dramatically improve your energy and performance. The basic practice involves optimizing your awareness and practice of good "recovery mechanisms"—those psychological and physiological recuperative periods such as sleep, vacations, and breaks in the day that provide your body and brain the chance to restore health, energy, and balance. Many businesspeople seem to suffer from a deep-seated Puritanical compunction that makes them feel guilty when they begin to get a little tired. But the fact is that your body and mind have a cyclical need for rest, just as they have a cyclical need for food and water. And taking time out for high-quality recuperation, like supplying yourself with nutritious food, is critical to maintaining an optimal state for performance.

Breaking into Busy Schedules

When I discuss the subject of breaks with businesspeople across the country, the response is predictable. Yes, they'd like to take time off to recuperate, during the day and throughout the year. But first of all, they would face the tacit disapproval on the part of their employer or coworkers. As one executive of a Fortune 500 company told me, "I know that taking breaks and honoring your vacation time is the intelligent thing to do, but the hectic pace here creates a source of peer pressure that says 'I'm working here until 7 P.M. on Friday night—why are you taking a break or leaving on Thursday for the weekend?' " And second, most people say they just can't afford to tack the time onto an already jam-packed schedule. In fact, the Professional Workforce Survey showed that while 79 percent believed that such breaks in the day would be valuable to their performance, 57 percent never or almost never take them.

Most people, however, have the situation backward. The fact that you are busy means that you should take *more* breaks, not fewer. That is, you should schedule a couple of brief but effective breaks in your workday to help you maintain a focused, energized state. In a high-pressure business environment, when you're expending a great deal of energy and concentration in tough, nerve-racking endeavors, a brief interval of downtime can dramatically improve your long-term health and your short-term performance. While withdrawing from work for a few minutes temporarily halts your output, good breaks can erase tension, engender optimism, focus the mind, and jump-start creative problem solving—changes that substantially increase your overall productivity. To put the matter in simplistic mathematical terms, why work for two hours at a slightly unfocused 75 to 80 percent when you can take a fifteen-minute interval of downtime and then work for an hour and forty-five minutes at a surging 100 percent?

Traditionally, many companies have opposed taking breaks, and many people have considered them a sign of weakness. With the shift to a business environment that demands more flexibility and better ideas, however, many people are changing their attitude. At Microsoft, it was never even an issue. Microsoft has always fostered an environment in which taking time to relax and clear your head is not just allowed, it's encouraged. "People at our company know it's part of their job to take an afternoon off to think a problem through—we encourage them to take off," says Jodi Hobbs, a marketing specialist at Microsoft's Phoenix office. Hobbs considers recovery breaks invaluable: while she doesn't formally schedule breaks into her day, she has a range of practices she follows to revitalize her energy, mood, and thinking.

When she feels the need to briefly rest her mind, for example, Hobbs will put a CD in her computer's CD player and go through e-mails or clean up her computer files. If she's upset, she takes a more complete time-out: "I will put my head down on my desk, close my eyes, and just breathe deep and think for a few minutes." And if she really feels a need for rejuvenation, Hobbs clears out of the office and goes for a hike on Camelback Mountain. "If something's bothering you, it gives you a chance to clear your mind, or if you just have an enormous amount to do, it gives you the chance to kind of regroup and organize it in your mind," Hobbs says. "I have a different perspective when I walk through the door again."

The CatchFire prescription for integrating recovery mechanisms into your schedule includes intelligently planning breaks in your day, performing relaxation exercises that restore your mental and physical health, getting adequate sleep, and indulging your needs for vacations and outside interests. And the great thing about many of these relaxation and recovery strategies is that you can achieve terrific results without dedicating much time or effort. At the office, you can perform simple, effective techniques, taking as little as 5 to 10 minutes, that will recharge your energy level and renew your outlook on life. And you don't have to disrupt the office by burning incense, standing on your head, or tapping kegs of barley brew. At its most basic, the procedure involves putting down your work, holding your calls, closing your eyes, and taking some deep diaphragmatic breaths. Whether you're busy or not, the results are too good to pass up.

The new approach that a number of athletes are taking toward their training offers an instructive example of the effectiveness of realigning your work patterns. Many individual athletes such as tennis players are eschewing extensive, exhausting practices for shorter, more tightly structured sessions interspersed with well-orchestrated periods of recovery. Rather than practicing long hours for the sake of practicing long hours, as some were prone to do, they mix up focused drilling with periods of rest or other modes of training: strength exercises, video analysis, visualization, and participation in other sports (low-risk activities—ski jumping and pole vaulting are out). The results? Not only do most report far fewer injuries, but they feel that a schedule of more intense, enthusiastic workouts and well-defined recovery periods is both more effective and more fun.

The Cycles of Work and Recovery

Part of the reason that paying attention to recovery periods is so essential is that many people in today's business world are literally pushing themselves to the limit. The Japanese, known for exhausting work schedules, have gone so far as to coin a term for the outbreak of fatal exhaustion that has caused a number of young executives to drop dead at their desk. They call it *karoshi*, which means "death by overwork." After seeing an alarming rise in overwork fatalities a few years ago, Japanese medical authorities published a list of the leading warning signals of *karoshi*. Among them are working high-pressure jobs without breaks; working extremely long hours that interrupt normal cycles of rest; and not taking time off for holidays or other breaks.

It's easy to understand how periods of rest—whether breaks in a day or vacations throughout the year—get squeezed out of hectic schedules. But constantly maintaining a furious pace violates one of the governing principles of health and vitality: the body operates according to a cycle in which periods of activity are followed by periods of rest and recovery. You work, expend energy, grow tired, and rest; and then, refreshed and rejuvenated, you

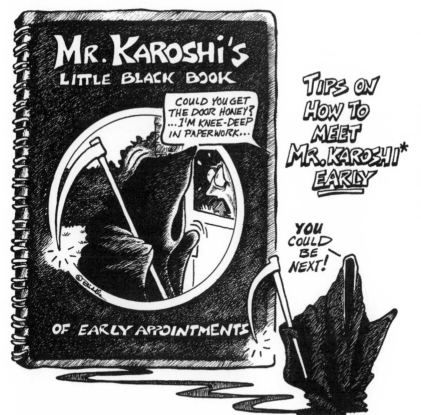

*KAROSHI – JAPANESE TERM FOR DEATH BY OVERWORK

can return to your endeavors. This basic cyclical rhythm, in fact, runs through all of nature. Seasonal blossoming, the recurring need for food and sleep, the regular inhaling and exhaling of breath, and the pulsations of the heart all illustrate the cyclical nature of life. Obviously, there are times when your work doesn't correspond with these rhythms, and you just can't break away. But far from being expendable, the low parts of the cycle—the downtimes or periods of inactivity—constitute an essential part of the processes that create energy and health.

As leading researchers such as Dr. Hans Selye, Dr. Herbert Benson, and Dr. Ernest Rossi have discovered, continually depriving yourself of recovery periods enfeebles your body and brain. In periods of recovery, the body undergoes an interval of self-service in which muscles are rebuilt, growth hormones are released, disease-fighting cells of the immune system are replenished, and the stock of neurotransmitters that facilitate mental alertness and concentration are replaced. Battling through a day of anxiety-producing pressures, however, chronically triggers the "fight or flight" response, which denies your body and mind these vital periods of restoration. With recovery mechanisms such as sleep, the effect is immediately apparent: cutting into your nighttime slumber results in greater irritability and fatigue. But similar disturbances in mind and body result from disregarding the need for breaks throughout the day, or neglecting relaxation exercises, vacations, and interests outside of work. In fact, concentrated activity without pause turns out to be one of the predominant mechanisms by which stress negatively impairs your health.

The Einstein Walkabout

In addition to helping you avoid the negative effects of chronic stress, though, practicing good recovery strategies prepares you to thrive in a tough business environment by elevating your attitude and the quality of your thinking. You could afford to be inflexible, uncooperative, or mentally sluggish if you worked a repetitive job, as most people did a couple of decades ago. But when you're creating innovative products, totally redesigning the processes of your department, or working on a marketing campaign that has to quicken a customer's pulse, then bumbling through the project with shallow enthusiasm and half-baked ideas won't cut it. You need to reach a higher plane of thought and action.

And this is where a high-powered "attitude adjustment" period can redeem you. A brief period of downtime gives you a chance to turn inward for reflection, introspection, and wonder. A haven from the surrounding chaos and the constant mental exertion of your work, downtime gives you space to clear your head, breathe, and temporarily substitute your worm's-eye perspective for a bird's-eye view. Physiologically, the brain naturally transmits more calming, creativity-inspiring alpha waves during recovery periods. In addition, the right hemisphere of the brain—the one that specializes in pattern recognition—is more active throughout these periods, suggesting that relaxation breaks offer an excellent opportunity to reframe and reconceptualize your problems.

Fine-tuning a relaxation break to your schedule and needs—perhaps having a banana and going through a 10-minute muscle relaxation exercise every afternoon at 3 o'clock—can break the grip of tension and recalibrate inefficient activity. Accessing a deeper level of calmness, focus, and creativity, you can set yourself back to work in full command of your powers. Albert Einstein said that break periods were a great inspiration to his thinking. He didn't get his great ideas when he was working at the blackboard; he got them when he was out walking around and eating an apple.

To describe the process as simply as possible, I often use the analogy of automobile maintenance, in this case for a high-performance race car. During daily races, rigorous driving at top speeds consumes fuel, depletes resources, and pushes the systems of the car to the limit. Periodically, the car has to have a break—that is, a pit stop—to refuel, replenish reserves of oil, and replace well-worn tires. Pit stops keep the car running at maximal levels throughout the race, just as periodic breaks help you maintain your optimal energy and concentration at work. At the end of the day, the car is put through a more complete maintenance stop, replacing fluids, lubricating various components, and retuning parts of the engine—a process similar to the more complete rest and recovery period of sleep. And finally, a few times a year the car needs to undergo a more complete servicing—possibly an overhaul—with parts rebuilt and systems revamped. The occasional overhaul parallels the more thorough restoration period of a vacation, an interval in which you more fully revive your body, mind, and spirit.

Dancing to a Faster Rhythm

Comparing the pace of life in today's business world with people's habits in different cultures and times affords a better perspective on how we have historically integrated work and leisure. Not surprisingly, such a comparison reveals that life in the late-twentieth-century United States moves much faster than life in the vast majority of other societies. And it reinforces the notion that, since we drive ourselves harder than most civilizations would consider natural or reasonable, we should establish and vigilantly guard our periods of rest and recuperation.

Harvard economist Juliet Schor, in *The Overworked American,* describes how our society ranks with the very top in terms of time devoted to work. In the fourth century, Schor says, the Roman calendar listed 175 public festival days per year—a number that stayed fairly constant in the West through medieval and Renaissance times. (It turns out that the Pilgrims, those relentlessly industrious folk, cut approximately fifty of the holidays from the American work schedule.) Many modern-day primitive societies put in a very leisurely workweek. !Kung bushmen, for instance, work only two and a half days per week, at an average of six hours per day. The Kapauku of Papua New Guinea busy themselves with labor about every other day. Of course, none of these past or present societies enjoys the standard of material comfort that contemporary industrialized nations do. But in terms of the ratio of work to leisure, people in today's business world carry an uncommonly heavy burden.

The current tempo of life has a further important difference from earlier times: it creates a life of seemingly perpetual motion, in which many people lack daily restorative periods of relaxation that almost all previous societies enjoyed. As Dr. Herbert Benson points out, all major religions embrace some sort of daily practice that quiets the mind and calms the body. In the past, people generally performed these exercises by situating themselves in a quiet environment, assuming a specific position, and repeating a certain word, phrase, or thought. Christianity, for example, has various periods of prayer throughout the day; Buddhism has the practice of meditation; Taoists engage in a diverse array of yogic breathing techniques; and the Islamic tradition includes designated times for ritual chants or prayers. Although most practitioners were unaware of it, these exercises had a dramatic physiological response: they produced a slowed, peaceful state of recovery that counteracted the effects of negative stress and promoted health and recuperation. Of course, many people still pray and meditate. But for most, the practice is neither as regular nor as extensive as it was for past societies. Viewed from this perspective, some sort of daily relaxation ritual is conspicuously absent from the average routine of modern life.

I don't mean to imply that the human body isn't capable of hard work (it is) or that your work can't be enormously entertaining (it can and by all means should be). But to maintain the peak levels of energy, focus, and calmness necessary to thrive in such conditions, you have to practice a routine of rest and relaxation. A good place to start is to orchestrate your workday around your body's natural cycles of energy.

Orchestrating Breaks Throughout the Day

When you're climbing Mount Everest, the grueling physical exertion and stifling lack of oxygen leave you little choice: you have to take periodic breaks. The world-renowned mountaineer Ed Viesturs, when leading a group up the mountain, strictly enforces a 15-minute "maintenance stop" after every hour of hiking—a period in which climbers sit down, stretch, drink, snack, and gear up their bodies and minds for another arduous push. Forsaking such breaks, especially at higher elevations, can induce dizziness, loss of concentration, exhaustion, and even more dire physical and mental breakdowns.

The consequences of extended exertion aren't quite so severe when you're sitting in your office—warm, dry, and somewhere near sea level. But the principle still applies. As research shows, after every hour and a half to two hours of focused activity, your body and brain experience a downturn in performance. Most likely, if you look at a typical day, you'll find that your energy level roughly adheres to such a pattern: after dedicating a couple of hours to a sales proposal or a rapid-fire series of phone calls, your body signals that it needs a time-out. You feel an urge to walk around, stretch, get a snack or a drink, or just take your mind off work for a few minutes. Overriding this desire on occasion won't prompt a nosedive in your performance; but disregarding the need at crucial times, or on a regular basis, will often cause you to work at considerably lower levels of vitality and focus. It will promote the all-too-common state of semialertness and lukewarm enthusiasm. On the other hand, observing a break schedule that corresponds to the natural energy cycles of your body—and making the most out of these periods with relaxation exercises—maximizes your performance over the day.

The science underlying the periodic or rhythmic behavior of the body and brain centers around what is called the basic-rest-activity-cycle (BRAC). The basic-rest-activity-cycle describes how many of the physiological functions of the body—including certain hormone and neurotransmitter release, patterns of cerebral activity, and even genetic processes at the molecular level—take place on a periodic basis. For example, each evening the body secretes the hormone melatonin to promote sleep and facilitate growth. To complicate the picture slightly, these periodic changes are governed by two different cycles or rhythms: *circadian rhythms* and *ultradian rhythms.* Circadian rhythms, simply put, direct the changes in the body and brain that lead to states of sleep or wakefulness. Ultradian rhythms describe the more subtle but still powerful shifts in hormone release and physiological functions that occur, on average, eight to twelve times a day. It is the ebb and flow of these rhythms that set the "energy cycles" of your body and mind throughout the day, and therefore dictate the best times to schedule breaks.

Interestingly, government laboratories blindly stumbled onto the phenomenon of ultradian rhythms when investigating the source of human error in on-the-job accidents. Researchers found that activity, performance, memory, and reaction time corresponded to regular periods throughout the day. More specifically,

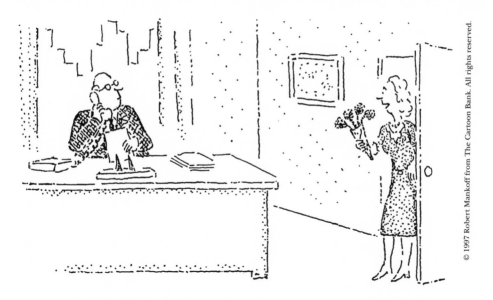

"Sorry to interrupt, Mr. Barksdale, but you're scheduled to take time out to smell the roses."

their studies revealed that people operate with high levels of performance for an hour and a half to two hours, and then experience a decline in functioning for approximately 20 minutes—a time in which a disproportionately large number of accidents occurred. From this initial discovery, scientists from a wide variety of specialties have found many other bodily functions that conform, in some manner, with this rhythm.

Dr. Ernest Rossi, the author of *The Twenty-Minute Break* and *The Psychobiology of Mind-Body Healing*, is the leading authority on ultradian rhythms. From years of research and clinical experience, Rossi has found that aligning your work with these activity cycles contributes greatly to your health and performance. "During the first hour or so of this rhythm, we swing upwards on a wave of heightened physical and mental alertness and energy, our skills, memory, and learning ability at their peak for dealing with the world around us," Rossi says. You stay at this peak level for another 30 to 60 minutes—for a total of an hour and a half to two hours of concentrated activity. At that point starts a downturn: "Then, for the next fifteen to twenty minutes, we swing down to a performance low at which we usually feel like taking a rest. In this phase, many of our systems of mind and body attempt to turn inward for a period of heightened healing and recharging for renewed endeavor." Rossi calls this downtime the "ultradian healing response," emphasizing how the physiological processes in this 20-minute period mend the wear and tear on the body.

The basic rule defined by these peaks and troughs of performance is simple, and almost intuitive: for every one and a half to two hours of work, you can optimize your energy and performance by taking a 15- to 20-minute break.

BREAKING UP YOUR DAY

If you put in a normal workday, scheduling breaks to accord with your ultradian rhythms is relatively simple. The schedule naturally coincides with many formally instituted break periods because, at least in part, these break periods were established at times when people naturally feel a downturn. Assuming that you arrive at work at 8:00 to 8:30 A.M., you should take a midmorning break, of 15 to 20 minutes, at around 10:00 A.M. Your second break comes at lunchtime—at noon or slightly after. And then, after another hour and a half to two hours of dedicated activity, your midafternoon break should fall at about 3:00 P.M. After work, the breaks become less important for the reason that, even if you have to make dinner for your family and attend to other household work, you don't have to exert focused attention under stress, and thus don't have a great need for restoration. If you do work late, then continue to follow the rule—15 to 20 minutes of downtime for every 90 to 120 minutes of work.

What should you do during your break? I'll shortly discuss a number of quick, effective activities—from stretching to snacking to walking—that you can use to optimize your 15- to 20-minute recovery period. But the chief directive is a simple one: cease intensive action. Don't negotiate your salary, don't call an angry customer, and don't plunge into the most critical, complicated aspect of your current assignment. Left to its own devices, the body will induce the biological changes that restore energy and strength. All you have to do is recognize your body's cue to lay off the heavy stuff, sit back, and relax.

Fortunately, ultradian rhythms are flexible and responsive. Evolution prepared us to override our slow periods if an emergency threatened. So although every ultradian healing response helps maintain peak levels of energy and focus, you should take breaks according to your individual temperament, the nature of your work, and your office environment. Some people find that they don't need a midmorning break. Others feel that a 10-minute interval is all they need to clear their mind and renew their enthusiasm. In fact, most people find that two or three significant breaks a day (which includes one at lunch) sufficiently recharge their batteries. As always, the number one rule is to tune in to what your body is telling you, and let this advice dictate your recovery schedule.

At CIGNA Insurance Company, rest and recovery periods are winning an impressive following. The Wellness Center in the 5,000-person office in Philadelphia has masterminded Fast Break, a program that teaches simple, stress-busting tools to employees in workplace settings. Here's how it works: an instructor from the Wellness Center goes to a specific meeting or department at an appointed time and conducts a 5-, 10-, or 15-minute session consisting of a combination of deep breathing, active stretching, and guided visualization exercises. So, for example, when Lisa Alvarez, the assistant manager of CIGNA's Human Resource Division, was hosting an important and potentially tense meeting to introduce the new head of the department, she scheduled a Fast Break for the middle of the afternoon. "The day was long and intense because we were working through a process that allowed people to ask some pretty difficult questions," Alvarez says. Her feeling that the group would need recharging in the middle of the serious discussion was right on target: "The break was right when everyone was tired and a little bit brain-dead, and there was a lot of tension in the room." A quick and well-designed recovery period, however, transformed the atmosphere of the meeting.

Led by an able instructor, the group revved up with a mini aerobics class—some easy movement such as marching in place and conga line dancing—for 7$\frac{1}{2}$ minutes. Then, sitting back down in their chairs for another 7½ minutes, they went through a progressive muscle relaxation exercise set to calming music. For Alvarez, the 15-minute interval worked wonders: "It really forced me to stop and think about how I was doing mentally and physically. It helped provide tension release and it helped get me focused back on being productive for the rest of the day." The rest of the group, she reports, found it equally invigorating: "Everybody loved it. They thought it was a perfect way to reenergize. It put everyone back in a productive frame of mind." And the break didn't merely improve the company's dance moves or harmony with the universe; the meeting, Alvarez says, was unquestionably more effective than it would have been otherwise.

THE BREAKING POINT

The midafternoon break, for many people, is the most crucial. In fact, researchers call the period around 3:00 P.M. the "breaking point." Ultradian and circadian rhythms simultaneously drop at this time, and as a number of tests reveal, natural levels of alertness, energy, and performance sink to one of the lowest points in the day. Experiments involving sleep, for example, demonstrate that when secluded from daylight, clocks, and calendars, and allowed to sleep whenever they want, subjects choose to sleep twice each twenty-four-hour period—once at night for seven or eight hours, and once in the midafternoon for a short nap. Accidents on the job also seem to correspond with these regular cycles of activity and alertness, falling primarily into two periods—the first and most pronounced from 1 A.M. to 8 A.M., and the second during the period from 2 P.M. to 6 P.M. In short, while nightly sleep is the most substantial recovery period, the body and mind hunger for a rest interval in the afternoon as well. Instead of fighting and dragging your way through this ebb in the cycle, you're much better off heeding the call for a break and giving your body the recuperation it needs. Refreshed and refocused after a brief respite, you can finish the day with a flourish of productive activity.

How do you use the activity and rest principle when working long hours under pressure? To work most effectively, you have to evaluate what you have to accomplish, know your individual energy cycles and stamina, and plan the attack in a way that best utilizes your resources. Of course, you can't take the rest of the day off every time you feel tired or stuck; converting your projects and goals into reality sometimes requires long, intense sessions in which you just have to grind the work out. But it's important to know when you can take a break, do some deep breathing, revitalize yourself, and churn out your work—and when you're better off just calling it a day.

While I've always believed that people have vast untapped resources, you have to recognize when you have reached the point at which your focus, judgment, and sanity have abandoned you. Slogging forward at such a time invites frustration and failure. It's not brave so much as stupid. And if done habitually, it can impair your health, sap your confidence, and create an enduring sense of defeat. As Dan Robertson, the CFO of Printing Industries of America, says, "Occasionally, I'll have someone tell me, 'I can't work on that project right now because my mind is mush.'" Robertson doesn't take that as a sign of weakness, but as a sign of wisdom: "I like that. Because I don't want somebody on the job who's not up to it. It'd be like an airline pilot saying 'My vision isn't too good, but I think I can make it.' I mean, thanks, but I'll wait here and catch the next flight."

Maximizing Your Recovery Periods

The following activities will help you get the optimal benefit from your breaks:

TAKE A BREATHER

In the chapter on awareness, I discussed what a simple and powerful tool breath control is. But to recapitulate, taking deep breaths from the base of your stomach relaxes the body and focuses the mind. And it's extremely flexible: whether you're in a meeting, at your desk, in an airplane, or in your car, you can instantly and easily engage in a deep-breathing session.

Thousands of breathing exercises exist, aimed at inducing a variety of effects. But the simplest versions are all that are necessary to enhance your energy and mood. Basically, the process involves breathing slowly and deeply from the diaphragm. If possible, start by closing your eyes (except when driving) and sitting with your head up, back straight, and muscles relaxed. To ensure that you are breathing from the diaphragm, consciously push your stomach out as you inhale, putting your hand on your stomach to feel it moving out. Inhale through the nose—slowly, calmly, evenly— for a count of 4, and then exhale for another four counts, letting out all feelings of tension and worry. Notice the wave of relaxation washing over your entire body as you breathe. Feel yourself becoming more calm, focused, and energized. Continue the process for the 2, 10, or 20 minutes that you can spend on the exercise.

The number of counts is flexible. Some people prefer to use a count of 6 or 8, and some breathe without bothering to count. Additionally, many people advocate breathing out through the mouth. Experiment with these variations and find what works for you. The exact method matters little; the most important rule is to use whatever technique feels most natural and comfortable.

Many people find consciously focusing on deep breaths to be the single most valuable method of relaxation. The simple act of regulating your breath will help you not only relax when you need a break but also regain a sense of calmness and control in any situation. As Chuck Inman, Group Product Director at Alcon Surgical, says, "One of the most effective things I do when I'm tired or tense is just to take a couple moments of quiet time, and do some deep breathing." Sometimes, Inman told me, he'll take a few minutes to breathe deeply while sitting in his car, before going in to visit a customer.

MUSCLE OUT TENSION

Mental and emotional tension manifest themselves in the body. When feeling anxious, most people carry their tension in the back, shoulders, and neck. Fortunately, the reverse is also true:

physical relaxation of the body creates calmness in the mind. In fact, some studies show that it is simply impossible to be physically relaxed and mentally anxious at the same time. By engaging in certain muscle relaxation exercises, you can use this relationship to ease feelings of anxiety and create a positive mood.

Progressive relaxation is a method in which you alternately tense and relax the various muscle groups throughout your body. Most methods start with the toes and move up to the head; but if you're working with limited time, you may want to confine your exercise to your back, neck, and shoulders, or wherever you're most prone to feel tense. While lying down with your eyes closed is the ideal position, the exercise is effective when you do it sitting in your chair at the office.

To start, gradually tense the muscles in one muscle group—say, your shoulders—and then hold them tight and flexed for about 10 seconds. As you hold them, notice that this sensation is the feeling of tension, and notice that you have control over it. Then, after holding the muscles tight for several seconds, slowly let go of the tension, gradually releasing all tautness until your muscles are completely relaxed. It's important not to "try to relax," because this implies effort and exertion, which can lead you to tense up. Instead, adopt a passive, "let-it-happen" mentality. Once you've reached complete relaxation in your muscles, again note that this is the feeling of relaxation, and realize that you have control over it.

A great muscle-relaxation session includes tensing and relaxing your toes, lower legs, upper legs, arms, lower abdomen, upper abdomen, shoulders, neck, jaw, face, and scalp. But a succinct exercise involving three or four of these muscle groups can afford you a deep sense of calmness and comfort.

TAKE A WALK

Studies conducted by Robert Thayer, author of *The Origins of Everyday Moods,* show that as little as a 5-minute walk can significantly increase energy and reduce tension. Especially for the multitudes who spend the majority of their workday glued to their desk and chair, going for a brief stroll can be a perfect activity for your break.

Try to walk outside, in a park or down a pleasant street. If that's not possible, even a walk through your building or up and down the stairs provides a healthy break from sitting at your desk. Breathe deeply, draw your shoulders back, and stride with a loose, confident, comfortable gait. And don't think about your job; allow your mind, as well as your feet, to wander away from your work.

HAVE A SNACK

If you feel hungry, have a light, healthy snack during your break. Having a piece of fruit, half of a bagel, or something low in fat and calories keeps your blood sugar level balanced, which helps maintain a positive mood and mental focus.

Having a drink of water is also a great idea. The body needs six to eight glasses of water a day to stay optimally hydrated, a quota few people fulfill. I make it a habit to visit the water cooler every time I take a break.

SHIFT TO A DIFFERENT, LESS DEMANDING ACTIVITY

If you can't take a total break from work, one way to get partial benefit from the ultradian restorative processes is to occupy yourself with different and less intensive work. Alternating your tasks allows you to use a different part of your brain. Slowing down enables you to enjoy a more relaxed pace for a while. So switch to a simple job for 10 minutes to facilitate at least some relief and regeneration.

If you've been on the phone all morning, check your e-mail or do some light reading. If you've been staring at a computer screen for a couple of hours, go talk to some colleagues. Keep a list of easy, routine tasks you can do when you need to downshift from high-intensity work.

LISTEN TO MUSIC

Music—particularly slow, soothing music—is an ideal accompaniment to a recovery period. Any music that you like will help put you in a positive mood. But even better, a number of relaxation tapes and CDs, specially designed to entrain your brain to alpha waves (which are associated with feelings of calmness and comfort), can facilitate a positive, relaxed state of mind.

In some office environments playing music might be unsuitable. But if you're at home, in the car, or if you have a Walkman, I highly recommend augmenting your relaxation sessions with music.

While I don't rigidly schedule breaks in my day, I almost always follow the prescribed outline of midmorning, lunch, and afternoon recovery periods. My midmorning breaks tend to be brief. I normally eat a piece of fruit or part of a low-fat energy bar, fill up my glass of water, and take a few minutes to look over a newspaper. For lunch, I ordinarily go out, walk to one of the nearby restaurants, and have a healthy, relaxed meal. Midafternoon breaks are the most necessary for me. At the minimum, I'll take 10 minutes and put my work down. A couple of times per week, our staff meets in the main room to listen to a relaxation tape and do some deep breathing. (I know our mailman thinks we're great people, but the couple of times he's come in to find us like this no doubt caused him to wonder just what the hell we really do.) Additionally, I have a light snack and another refill of water.

Some days, my recovery periods are brief. On other days—if I have a busy schedule or I've just gotten home from a long trip— they might be extensive. But particularly when I'm doing some reading, writing, and program-design work that requires top levels of concentration and creativity, I depend heavily on these recovery periods, not only for renewed energy, but for fresh perspectives and novel ideas. Often, I'll emerge with a different tack on a project, or a new angle on a problem.

Block Off Your Breaks

"I see people become slaves to their own work schedules, and won't take a break during the day," one executive told me. "They work through lunch and then at three o'clock run out to get a hamburger." Obviously, a surgeon isn't going to take a break in the middle of a long operation, and a Wall Street trader isn't going to sit down for a breathing exercise in the middle of the trading floor. Everyone, on occasion, has to work through a half-crazed day during which even a 15-minute recovery period is 15 minutes too long.

But when most people say they don't have time for a break, it's because they fail to take control of their work schedule. If spontaneously fitting them in yields no more than a couple of breaks per week, then more severe methods are in order. Block off 15 minutes in your Day-Timer. Transfer calls to voice mail. Leave the office if you need to. But make taking breaks a ritual, and realize that they are a necessary pit stop that will enhance, not detract, from your productivity. Call them a "performance break" if you feel guilty about not keeping constantly busy. But try a relaxation session and see if it doesn't leave you rejuvenated and sharp.

Debbie Veney Robinson, a spokesperson for CIGNA, says the Fast Break program is especially popular with individuals who say they don't have time for a break but by all outward appearances desperately need one. In fact, when these people participated in some form of tension-taming, energy-enhancing exercise through the Wellness Center, almost all found it invigorating and enjoyable. As Robinson says, "People say that it helps them so much to refocus, to leave what they are doing for a minute so they can get recharged and come back at it with a clearer mind and more energy. People love it."

Total Quality Sleep

"Most Americans no longer know what it feels like to be fully alert," says Dr. William Dement, Director of Stanford University's Sleep Research Center, in a *Time* magazine article. "They go through the day in a sort of twilight zone; the eyes may be wide open, but the brain is partly shut down."

From discussions with audiences across the country, I'm amazed at how many people just accept poor sleep and the consequent downturn in energy and mood. Sleep is the number one recovery mechanism, the process that most thoroughly restores our psychological and physiological vitality after the strain and exertion of a long, busy day. Yet most people don't sleep long enough or well enough. In fact, over 100 million Americans say they have occasional problems sleeping. Over half of the respondents of the Professional Workforce Survey reported "fair" to "poor" quality of sleep. A comprehensive report by the National Commission on Sleep Disorders Research stated the problem definitively: "One thing is absolutely certain in America: The quality and quantity of sleep obtained are substantially less than the quality and quantity needed." The commission also said that companies lose a staggering $15.9 billion in productivity every year because of people nodding off at their desks.

Promising new studies, however, show you how to optimize the restoration and refreshment you get from your nightly rest, thereby enhancing your energy, mood, and performance.

A variety of experiments on sleep's effect on performance have reported different and sometimes contradictory results. Some studies indicate that sleep deprivation can detract from performance by as much as 30 percent; others show that one night of total sleep loss has little impact on your ability to function. But the consensus is that reduced sleep, at the very least, leads to increased irritability and fatigue. The majority of Professional Workforce Survey respondents felt that sleep deprivation takes its toll: 71 percent said that it negatively affects their performance at work the next day. In my seminars, I consistently find that the majority of people say the day after a poor night of sleep is marked by trouble paying attention in meetings (especially boring ones), reduced ability for mental concentration and creativity, and a general state of lethargy.

Physiologically, sleep is the repair shop of the body and brain. Like the ultradian healing responses that take place during the day, certain intervals of sleep initiate a number of restorative

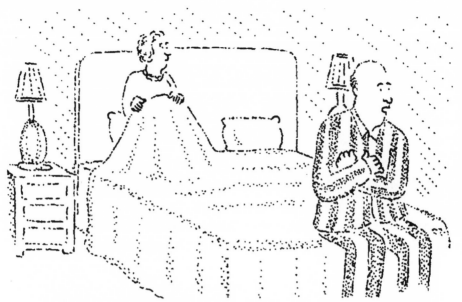

"How can I sleep when people in other time zones are already up and making money?"

biological processes. In addition to more completely rebuilding your muscle tissue, bones, cell walls, immune system cells, and neurotransmitters, some periods of deep sleep discharge important hormones such as the human growth hormone, which plays a major role in the growth and vitality of the body. Losing sleep from insomnia or late nights of work prevents you from experiencing these vital recovery processes—which leaves you much less likely to work at high levels of energy, focus, and productivity.

QUANTITY OF SLEEP

So how much sleep should you get? Sleep requirements vary widely, depending on the individual. For most people—about two-thirds of the population—seven to eight hours per night is optimal. Others need more than eight hours to feel energetic and alert throughout the day. Almost 20 percent of the population, however, can function effectively with six hours of sleep—and some people can get away with even less. I was always amazed at the sleep habits of my friend the late Marshall McLuhan, the author and media expert, who slept only four hours a night (an amount he supplemented with a couple of 20-minute naps throughout the day), but remained ever witty, creative, and brilliant.

As usual, you have to determine from experience how much sleep is best for you. If you don't have a sense of how much sleep you need, use seven to eight hours as a general rule, and experiment with the effects of sleeping more or less until you find an optimum number of hours. (And take into consideration that this number will vary according to your daily patterns of behavior—you need more rest after taxing days.) But don't feel guilty about not sleeping for eight hours if you feel sufficiently rested and sharp with less.

QUALITY OF SLEEP

Recent research has concentrated more on the *quality* of sleep, and how it affects your biochemistry, energy, and mood. To see firsthand what sleep studies were talking about when they described the various factors of sleep, I visited a sleep apnea clinic to observe problem sleepers. While that doesn't sound like a rollicking night out, watching the process of sleep was surprisingly interesting. One of the subjects who was "asleep" tossed, turned, and twitched hundreds of times in a two-hour period. Constant readouts of brain waves, muscle tension, breathing rate, blood pressure, and body temperature allowed us to follow his and other subjects' progress through various stages of light and deep sleep. The change in brain-wave frequencies, in particular, was intriguing: as a subject moved from deep sleep to light sleep, the mechanical arm tracing the waves would advance from slow, steady curves to short, irregular, sometimes frenzied patterns. The experience hammered home the point that sleep is an active process, and a wide discrepancy exists between solid, revitalizing sleep and restless, agitated sleep.

Sleep researchers divide sleep into five stages. Stage one is the lightest stage of sleep, a twilight state of consciousness that marks the transition between wakefulness and sleep. As sleep deepens through stages two and three, brain-wave frequencies and many bodily processes slow down until they reach their lowest and most relaxed point in stage four. After spending anywhere from a few minutes to an hour in stage four sleep, you enter rapid eye movement, or REM, sleep, the state in which dreaming occurs. Every 90 to 120 minutes (following the same ultradian rhythm that operates during wakefulness), or about four or five times per night, you cycle down from stage one sleep to stage four, then back up for an episode of REM sleep.

Optimizing your sleep consists of maintaining the regularity of these cycles, and even more important, increasing the amount of time you spend in deep sleep (stages three and four)—which is the period in which the most complete physiological restoration occurs. The following are some of the most effective strategies for beating insomnia and increasing the incidence of refreshing deep sleep.

1. *Get some aerobic exercise during the day.* Studies show that aerobic exercise helps you sleep better. In addition to reducing insomnia, working out helps you get up to 33 percent more deep sleep. One caveat: do your exercise at least two hours before going to sleep.

2. *Reduce your consumption of caffeine and alcohol.* Especially when you drink it in the afternoon or evening, caffeine can hurt your ability to sleep. And while alcohol can make you feel sleepy, having more than two drinks can interfere with sleep patterns, causing you to get less deep sleep.

3. *Perform relaxation exercises.* Anxiety is the primary cause of sleep problems. Deep breathing, muscle relaxation techniques, and visualization can help relax your mind and create the physiological changes that accompany sleep.

4. *Play music that promotes sleep.* Specially designed CDs entrain brain waves to the delta frequencies of deep sleep. The music calms you down and helps you drop off.

5. *Avoid sleeping pills.* Fewer and fewer sleep specialists prescribe sedatives. They induce more light sleep at the expense of deep sleep, and they create a dependence on pills

rather than addressing the real problem. If you take them now, gradually eliminate the habit (possibly with the help of a physician).

6. *Establish regular hours of sleep.* Go to bed and get up at about the same time every day. The process helps produce a consistent circadian rhythm, which helps you feel tired at the right time for sleep.

Since I'm on the road almost two hundred days a year giving workshops and presentations, I sometimes suffer at the hands of jet lag and time changes, and have trouble sleeping. Aware that this sleep deficit was robbing me of energy, I bought some tapes (mentioned in number four above) designed to entrain brain waves from wide-awake beta waves, to the light sleep of alpha waves, to the dreaming sleep characterized by theta frequencies, and finally to the deep sleep of delta waves. I do a muscle relaxation exercise for the first 10 or 12 minutes, and I'm usually asleep before the tape is finished.

What I Didn't Do on My Summer Vacation

Sixty-eight percent of executives don't go on a vacation during the year, or take only a part of their allotted time. Their primary reasons: "too short staffed" or "too many things going on right now."

Whether you're an executive or not, you may feel that getting ready to leave for a week or two and the huge pile of work to clean up after you get back make the whole event too stressful. In fact, stress researchers put "family vacations" as one of the most stressful events in people's lives—right up there with death and divorce. But good vacations are a vital recovery mechanism, and well orchestrated, they can totally renew your enthusiasm and perspective.

Neal Groff, owner and CEO of the Madison Group, a wealth transfer insurance company in Denver, religiously observes his vacation time. An avid traveler, Groff enthusiastically plans about two months' worth of time off each year. One month, he normally goes to Europe—last year it was France—where he gets a whole new perspective on life while "laughing a lot more, drinking some wine, cycling through Provence, and meeting people with a whole new value set." He spends the other month on the beach in Hawaii or Mexico, where he tends to take a more easygoing, relaxing, reflective break. In addition to the extended vacations, he frequently takes three-day weekends in the mountains to ski or hike. Many days, Groff will work for three or four hours, and then hit the slopes for a few runs. He says these breaks make all the difference in handling the high stress—including long hours and last-second flights—involved in running his business.

Not everyone, of course, can go to Europe for a month. But it's crucial to your freshness and vitality to take time off from work. Whether your job is stressful or not, you need time to get away. At a minimum, you can stay home to relax and renew yourself. My mother, for example, ran a small real estate company, and she didn't travel as much as just take time off from work. Her vacation time was in December, when she prepared an elaborate celebration around Christmas. No matter what was going on in the office, she was making cookies, planning parties, and assembling the 2,000 lights that adorned our house and trees. She usually found a way to both plan parties and sell houses around Christmastime; but if a conflict presented itself, Christmas won every time.

Highly preferable to staying home to do yardwork or fix the roof is to do something new and interesting. Use your time off as a chance to indulge your passions in life—scuba diving, camping, golfing, traveling, or whatever else they may be. Dan Robertson of the Printing Industries of America believes so much in vacations that in addition to his three weeks of vacation time, he takes an additional two weeks off unpaid to feed his appetite for taking ski trips and going to the beach. The point is almost self-evident, but participating in your favorite activities and exploring new places of interest enhance your overall enthusiasm for and enjoyment of life.

As CEO of the $28 billion Canada Life, David Nield is leading

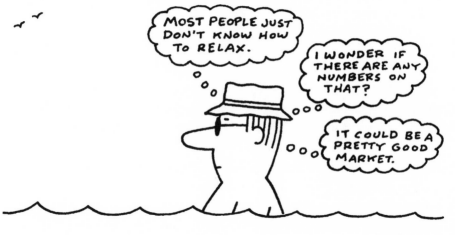

the company through restructuring, compensation adjustments, and a revamped recruitment policy. But without fail, he and his wife take time out for interesting, educational, adventurous vacations. When I worked with Canada Life last, the Nields were meticulously plotting out—with the help of a bewildering array of maps and books—a return trip to India. While neither is averse to beaches or leisure, they go on their vacations to learn and explore. I have no doubt that these trips refresh and renew Nield, and contribute significantly to the sense of focus, confidence, and vision he exhibits in the face of his demands.

Josef Pieper, one of the twentieth century's foremost philosophers, wrote in his essay *Leisure: The Basis of Culture* about vacations and leisure being not just a way to revive yourself for more work, but an invaluable opportunity to experience the joys and wonders of life. Leisure—the time to recover, relax, mull over new ideas and directions—expands your horizons and keeps fresh in your mind the sense of life as an adventure.

Get a Life

"You have to have a life outside of the business," says Jim Ruybal, Executive Vice President at United Artists. "I don't care what it is—family or spiritual, taking great vacations, or pets—as long as you have other dimensions so business doesn't become your life. If that happens, there's no safety valves to release the pressure." Jim Haymaker, Vice President at Cargill, couldn't agree more: "You're at risk if you're overwhelmingly focused on just one activity, unless it's an activity that you're absolutely in love with. I think playing a musical instrument, having hobbies, having sports you enjoy, having other cerebral activities like writing can be a great source of solace. Or just spending time with your kids and family. All those things are ways of shifting the focus and bringing perspective to your life."

While I don't mean to reduce family, friends, and personal avocations to mere "recovery mechanisms," devoting time to your relationships and outside interests is vital to maintaining top levels of health and enthusiasm. To people like Ruybal and Haymaker, engaging in a variety of outside activities is not just preferable, it's essential. These executives not only lead healthy, balanced lifestyles themselves, but they also consider such well-roundedness a critical factor in the people they choose for their teams. And so do the companies they work for. United Artists and Cargill, like most intelligently managed businesses, expect a lot from their people, but in return grant them a great deal of latitude with respect to their work schedules. The goal is to ensure that people have a life—or in other words, the opportunity to pursue interests outside work that keep them satisfied, vigorous, and fresh.

I don't begrudge anyone the opportunity to work passionately toward his or her dream, or labor diligently on a challenging project. But allowing work to crowd out other interests in life often heightens tension levels and narrows the mind. Concentrating exclusively on your job, like betting all your money on one race, causes you to lose a sense of proportion. With nothing else to divert you, problems loom larger. Worries grow more grave. And you tend to adopt a shortsighted mentality that diminishes your ability to think creatively, make good decisions, and handle high-pressure situations.

The same pressures, offset by a full docket of relationships, relaxation, and recreation, don't seem nearly as daunting. People who spend part of their week playing volleyball, going to concerts, fishing, or teaching their child to read tend to have a greater supply of psychological resources to cope with challenges at work—and even to enjoy them. Studies, in fact, have documented the correlation: whereas people who thrive on long hours of work tend to have varied interests and maintain close friendships, those who suffer from burnout owing to long hours of work tend to have few close friendships and limited outside interests. Having a life outside business allows you to absorb problems and defeats at work and roll with the punches. And more than that, taking part in activities you enjoy bolsters your general sense of fulfillment and exhilaration. When Paul Violassi of Softech Solutions plays a rousing game of hockey or when Kimberly McNally of Valley Medical Center pulls together a magnificent art exhibit, they renew their general excitement level in life.

Cross Training for the Brain

Pursuing outside interests also reinvigorates your thinking. Step 3 described how cross training—alternating the sports and exercises that you engage in—strengthens your muscular and cardiovascular systems much more effectively than repeatedly performing a single exercise. Pursuing outside interests is like cross training for the brain. Rather than devoting your thinking exclusively to work, spending time on recreational activities stretches your mind in new and different ways, limbering and sharpening your mental muscle. I don't mean that taking, say, a *tae kwon do* class will directly contribute to your plan for improved customer service. But such a practice will give you a chance to clear your mind and view the project with a fresh perspective. And further, somewhere in the creative, intermingling, cross-pollinating functions of the mind, a *tae kwon do* principle may provide the seed for a novel idea—a dazzling new approach to customer service that never could have sprouted from a mind planted over and over with the same crop. Samuel Johnson stated the matter definitively: "All intellectual improvement arises in leisure."

There isn't a formula to help you pursue your avocations and relationships. Basically, you just have to allocate time for them. Draw up a list of your favorite things to do, and vow to do them on a more regular basis. Don't do them when you get a chance, because a year will pass before you get one. Instead, commit yourself: sign up for a painting class, schedule next Saturday for a hike in the mountains, meet your friends for lunch every other Wednesday. A more enjoyable way to enhance your energy and mood is hard to find.

Working Smarter by Honoring Your Recovery Periods

Barry Triller, Executive Vice President at Mutual Life of Canada, aggressively pursues the creation of superior products, excellent customer service, and ever-increasing profits. And at the same time that he is working with his team to create such results, he is trying to reduce his hours at work.

Triller believes that if you don't work smarter—with top levels of energy and focus—you'll work longer to achieve the same or lesser results. He also believes in having a great life outside of business. A careful tracker of his time at work, he has gradually decreased his hours to an average of fifty to fifty-five hours per week, and says that "my actual goal is forty-eight hours of intense work per week." Does his awareness of time and vacations (he holds sacred his five weeks per year) pay off? Well, Mutual is among the top-producing insurance companies in Canada, Triller loves his job, and I can vouch that he has a hell of a lot of fun doing it.

I've seen it proved by many of the best performers: following the natural cycles of rest and recovery and honoring your needs for sleep and vacations will help you think more creatively, produce better quality, and enjoy life to the fullest.

CATCHFIRE TIPS FOR BREAKING UP STRESS AND FATIGUE

1. *Be aware of when your body and mind need reenergizing.* Give yourself permission to take a break.
2. *Build breaks into your schedule.* You need breaks every one and a half to two hours.
3. *Disengage and really relax.* Take a walk or use other relaxation techniques to sever your mind from work and create your own oasis of calm.
4. *When planning long meetings, don't forget the breaks.* Use the CIGNA Fast Break model to increase team energy and focus.
5. *Heed the "breaking point."* At 3 o'clock, take 15 minutes, have an apple, and do a diaphragmatic breathing exercise.
6. *Do a sleep audit.* If you're not sleeping well, change your habits and monitor the results.
7. *Plan adventurous vacations.* And take them.
8. *Shun one-dimensionality.* Constant work leads to dullness and/or burnout. Cultivate relationships and outside interests to foster energy and balance.

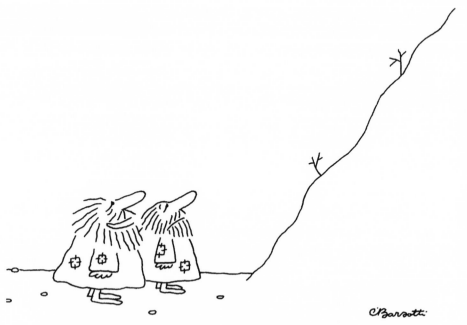

"Don't think of it as a hill, think of it as yet another opportunity to prove ourselves as worthy human beings."

STEP 5
Learning to Love Problems: The Challenge Response

Problems! We've got to have problems! We thrive on problems!
                    —Godfrey Hounsfield, inventor of the CT scan

A short time ago, Juan Rodriguez, a faculty member at the business school of the University of Colorado, asked me to give a presentation to one of his classes. As happens more often than I care to think about, we had trouble with the audiovisual equipment. With only a few minutes to go before starting time, we summoned the audiovisual people to help fix a problem in the video projection system.

As the students began filtering in, the a/v technicians, Rodriguez, and I were examining the possible sources of the problem. Random flickers of images on the screen raised our hopes, but the audiovisual specialists couldn't seem to get the system working. They said the problem was in the video cassette recorder, but they couldn't fix it now. Meekly apologizing, they put their hands in their pockets and left—presumably to return to more pressing duties.

Rodriguez, however, had reached a different diagnosis. He thought the trouble resided in the projection device on the ceiling in the center of the room. And without delay, he grabbed a chair, balanced himself on it rather precariously, and began investigating the projector. The scene left me feeling concerned for Rodriguez's safety, and slightly embarrassed for his brazenness: on his toes, arms stretched up, shirt untucked, fidgeting with the a/v system in the midst of an auditorium of students, he seemed to compromise his professional stature. But just as I started to suggest that I conduct the presentation without visual aids, he managed to figure out the problem and get the projector to work. Promptly replacing the chair, he strode to the front of the room and graciously introduced me. Problem solved.

The repair didn't represent an inspired act of genius. It didn't equal a triumph of justice throughout the land. But Rodriguez's approach to problem solving left a striking impression on me. Two audiovisual technicians—experts in their field, paid to take care of problems exactly like the one we had—resigned themselves after putting forth a meager effort. They tanked. Like foil figures in a Shakespearean play, they made more vivid Rodriguez's behavior: curious, unhesitant, determined, he attacked the problem without any complaints or the least sense of the project being beneath him. I suspect that this problem-solving aptitude partially fueled his brilliant success as one of the founding members of two prominent high-tech companies (StorageTek and Exabyte, both Fortune 1000 companies).

When presented with a problem, most people unthinkingly get upset or withdraw from the situation. As with Pavlov's dogs, their response is instant and automatic—a problematic stimulus provokes a bad mood in response. But to perform well in a world brimming with adversity, we need to reexamine our emotional response to difficult circumstances. Because despite their poor reputation, problems can provide an outstanding opportunity to elevate your levels of excitement and performance. By adopting Step 5 of the CatchFire program—the challenge response to problems—you can learn to use adversity to trigger a positive rather than a negative mind-set.

Thriving on Adversity

Problematic situations test your emotional mettle. When business is running smoothly and projects unfold according to plan, anyone can work with optimism and excitement. But the intrusion of a distressing setback—a hungry new competitor, a computer glitch that shuts down your system, or a failed round of negotiations—often disrupts enthusiasm and focus. Like a boulder plunging into the middle of a calm lake, a problem can dash mental and emotional equilibrium, and create a troubled, topsy-turvy state of mind. The prevailing climate of pressure and change already creates background tension; but a specific tangle or difficult development frequently goads you into a state of frustration, anxiety, or emotional withdrawal.

Maintaining top performance at work means you have to learn to effectively deal with problematic situations—to counteract the tendency to respond with worry or resignation, and instead consciously view adversity as a perfect occasion to engage in high drama, learn new knowledge and skills, and exercise grace under pressure. Everyone knows they don't think as astutely or work as skillfully when they are upset or disheartened. Reacting with dejection, anger, or worry—what I call the *tank* or *tension* responses—creates significant changes in your body and brain that undermine your ability to concentrate and make decisions. While reacting more positively frequently requires effort, you have to use the onset of a tough problem to transform yourself into a state of challenge. Immediately seize control of your thoughts—before the insidious cycle of doubts and worries can start—and begin investigating the ways the breakdown can be converted into a breakthrough. Acquiring this *challenge response* to problems dramatically improves your thinking and performance in the face of adversity.

The Professional Workforce Survey clearly reflects the power of the challenge response. In the survey, respondents who approach problems in a state of challenge and enthusiasm said they were far more effective in their jobs than those who didn't have such an attitude. Predictably, those who said they adopted an optimistic, energetic approach reported themselves less than half as likely to get frustrated or anxious as people who took a dimmer view of their obstacles. They also felt significantly lower levels of stress and higher levels of energy. In addition to reporting themselves to be superior performers overall, those who reacted to tough problems with enthusiasm and challenge said that they were much more likely (73 percent compared to 40 percent) to thrive when the pressure is on.

Focused on the Challenge

I've seen many teams run into trouble and quickly become demoralized. And I've seen several others fight, explore, and joke their way through thorny barriers, modeling the way you can use problems to grow stronger. One of the more impressive examples involved a project at United Artists.

A few years ago, United Artists decided to go into a new business and created the United Artists Satellite Theatre Network. Jim Ruybal of United Artists says that the company—dissatisfied that 80 percent of their movie theater income came from business that occurred from Friday afternoon to Sunday evening—was looking for new sources of revenue. Since they couldn't find a sizable audience during the midweek afternoons and evenings, the state-of-the-art theaters often sat nearly empty. In discussing this at an executive meeting, someone suggested a whole new approach: trying to tap into the huge corporate meeting market. After some research, they decided that the individual theaters could make excellent facilities for corporate training and other educational seminars. And then they took the idea a step further: why not link up the theaters nationwide via satellite in order to bring together audiences all over the country? In other words, someone like Bill Gates of Microsoft is videotaped giving a presentation to a group in Seattle, and Microsoft employees gathered in United Artists movie theaters around the country see him simultaneously on the big screen. (Microsoft has been one of the biggest early customers.)

With great planning and expense, they retrofitted theaters, put the satellites in the sky, and launched the Satellite Theatre Network. Despite the wondrous creation, however, the problem wasn't solved. As Ruybal (who heads the Satellite Theatre Network) says, "We all thought, 'Build it and they will come.' So we built it and for the first two years, not very many came." For most companies, the idea of going to a meeting in a movie theater was just too new and different. After the expense of creating the network, the group was feeling the pressure to make it produce. Ruybal recalls many meetings with the chief financial officer that were decidedly uncomfortable.

But throughout the struggle to successfully market the network and land deals, Ruybal remained focused on the excitement of the project: the terrific capability to serve as a vehicle for educational programs of all types and the vast opportunities of the network to deliver corporate training at a fraction of the price of a typical company meeting. He repeatedly said to himself: "What better way to facilitate corporate communication or launch a product than to get all employees involved in one place and let them see what's going on and feel like they are a part of it?" Despite the fact that they were not meeting corporate financial expectations, Ruybal and his team continued to accentuate their positive expectations for the network and persisted in taking an enthusiastic message to potential clients.

After working their way up a steep learning curve—soliciting a broad range of customers and refining their sales and marketing approach—the spirit of challenge and enthusiasm has prevailed. Now into their third year of the business, the Satellite Theatre Network is prospering. (And as Ruybal says, "The meetings with the CFO are a lot more fun.")

While the United Artists team offers a great example of the challenge response, contrasting the reaction of getting challenged with getting tense more vividly reveals the vast discrepancy between them. This difference is illustrated clearly in the story of the man and woman who decide to take a camping trip as a first date. As with many first dates, this one didn't turn out to be a match: by the end of a long day's hike, the couple found each other highly disagreeable and launched into an exchange of criticisms and complaints. But their bickering came to an abrupt halt when, in the midst of setting up the tent, they looked up and saw an enormous bear barreling down a mountain toward them. The man panicked, horrified at the sight of the ferocious beast. And he was even further disconcerted when he saw the woman calmly lacing up her running shoes. "I don't care how fast you think you can run," the man told her, "there's no way you're going to outrun that bear."

"I don't have to outrun the bear," the woman coolly responded. "I just have to outrun *you.*"

Problems vs. Predicaments

Before charging off to eradicate all traces of difficulty, however, it's important to determine what kind of quandary you are facing. The basic drive to hunt down a problem, get it in your sights, and squeeze the trigger is admirable. But some difficult circumstances are not given to neat resolution. As much as we would prefer that the universe unfold in a sensible manner, that conflicts have the absolute properties of a geometrical proof, and that all our problems dutifully submit to a four-step, ten-week timeline, reality is a far more complex affair. Attempting to step up and just lick a complex, troublesome situation sets you up for feelings of exasperation and futility. Instead, you have to learn to draw a distinction between a problem and a predicament.

A problem might not have a clear solution, but it has a set of parameters within which you can forge some sort of answer. Deciding how to handle a budget cut for your project, dealing with a public relations problem, figuring out how to tackle a totally new marketing assignment—these are problems. They probably require a great deal of work and a heavy dose of ingenuity. But in the end, as the deadline arrives, you submit your proposal or make your decision, and you're done.

A predicament, on the other hand, defies convenient analysis or precise categorization. Predicaments are indefinite and multifarious, even messy and muddled. We tolerate predicaments because while they inflict trouble, they also supply a source of tremendous worth. The concept is similar to the notion of a tragic flaw in classical or Renaissance drama. The term "tragic flaw" implies that if a certain personality trait were eradicated from the tragic hero, what remains would be a perfect person. The problem with this formulation lies in the fact that the "flaw" that leads to the hero's downfall is inseparably tied to his or her greatness. Hamlet, for example, suffered a terrible case of indecisiveness. But the core of his indecisiveness—his appreciation for the complexity of man and the mystery of existence—occasioned his brilliant soliloquies and noble stature.

Relationships represent the clearest example of a predicament. Even if you work with intelligent people, you often have to team up with someone you don't get along with. At its worst, this may compel a personnel shuffle. But if everyone makes substantial contributions, and the results are worth the trouble, then what you have is a predicament. As much as you should attempt to improve communications and adapt working styles to interact more effectively with people, you never really "solve" a problematic relationship. You do your best to ameliorate conflicts, but in the end you just live with the less than perfect circumstances.

I worked with a high-tech company a few years ago that faced just such a situation. Among its nine senior executives, the company had a director of operations and a director of marketing who couldn't stand each other. The CEO, however, liked them both and felt they were the two best people in the country for their respective jobs. So instead of getting rid of one of them, he moved the marketing department to a different floor in the building (the departments had previously shared the same one) and kept direct correspondence between the two executives to a minimum. The move didn't exactly create a state of harmony: from time to time, spats would break out and tempers would flare. But over the years that I worked with them, nothing happened that impeded the company's growth from $750 million to

$3 billion a year in revenue. By playing with the predicament in- stead of hastily taking action to solve the problem, the CEO ulti- mately navigated a very successful path.

As Richard Farson says in his book *Management of the Absurd,* "Dealing with a predicament demands the ability to put a larger frame around a situation, to understand it in its many contexts, to appreciate its deeper and often paradoxical causes and conse- quences." You can't use the distinction between problems and predicaments to excuse yourself from taking action or making tough decisions. But the first step to effective problem solving is to quickly assess the size and scope of your difficulty. Is it a prob- lem or a predicament? Either way, you have to face it with energy, confidence, and humor. But tilting toward a predicament as you would a problem can quickly lead to the frustration or anxiety that impairs your ability to perform.

Problem-Solving Responses

The *tank, tension,* and *challenge* responses constitute the dominant pattern of emotional reactions to problems. Obviously, there are more than three different emotional responses to problems. Within what I call the tension response alone is an array that spans from "slightly perturbed" to "royally pissed off," with "miffed," "irritated," "peeved," and "furious" all falling somewhere in between. My purpose isn't to provide an exhaustive classifica- tion of possible attitudes. Rather, it's to provide a framework that helps you easily identify what state of body and mind you are in when you're facing a tough set of circumstances. So instead of getting sucked unwittingly into a negative emotional state by a setback in your new product design or a discouraging quarter of sales results, this scheme helps you immediately recognize that you're anxious or tanking, and need to move into the challenge response.

The challenge response is the goal. To get there doesn't re- quire any complicated psychological tricks, but rather an en- hanced awareness of your usual responses to problems and the

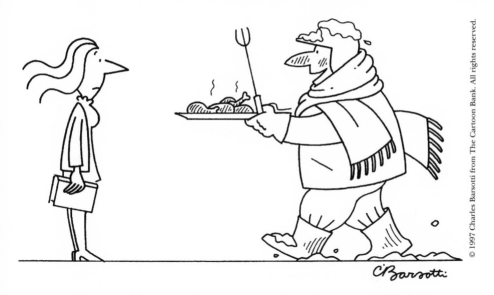

"There! And you said it was too lousy outside to barbeque."

kind of mental judo that enables you to shift from self-defeating emotional states to the more positive one of challenge. To reiterate, the element of awareness—the consciousness that you can decide how to react—plays an essential role in making this shift in mind-set. Awareness opens you up to the idea that, intrinsic in every moment, no matter how seemingly nerve-racking or discouraging, you have the chance to challenge yourself, create humor, or feel joy.

The analogy is somewhat crude, but you can almost picture yourself standing in front of some sort of vending machine, with large colorful squares representing your choices of problem-solving responses. You could, for instance, choose to hit the black one, and decide to duck the problem by willfully withdrawing all emotional investment and shrugging your shoulders in resignation. You could select the red one, and react with frustration and anxiety, tensing your muscles and raising your voice as you run through the potential catastrophes and vividly conjure up the ways this problem could lead to your ruin. Or you could choose the yellow square, and tackle the problem in a spirit of challenge, focusing on the opportunities to learn new skills and accomplish great things, and injecting a spirit of fun whenever possible.

THE TANK RESPONSE—
GOING THROUGH THE MOTIONS

To "tank" is to withdraw all emotional investment from the problem. The term comes from sports, and refers to instances in which an athlete—sensing defeat or so frustrated he doesn't care anymore—simply goes through the motions, indifferent to the outcome of the game. Tennis players in the tank response forgo any touch or finesse and unload on every ball—content if it goes in, unmoved if it doesn't. Basketball players neglect to move the ball around and set up plays, instead quickly shooting ill-advised outside shots. When tanking, players emotionally disengage themselves; their hearts aren't in the game. They don't play to fight their way back into the game, but to get it over with as quickly as possible.

Undoubtedly, you recognize parallel emotional responses at work. Most commonly, tanking occurs at times when you feel overwhelmed or exhausted (by some corollary of Murphy's Law, pernicious problems tend to strike at the most inopportune moments). In these cases, adversity doesn't arouse your innate response to fight or to flee—which is a reaction that requires effort and exertion. Instead, it arouses a response of less certain evolutionary heritage: the desire to lie down and hope the problem goes away. Whether rooted in weariness, frustration, or cynicism, the underlying attitude conveyed by word, posture, and behavior is "Screw it, I'm over this."

Tanking's effect on problem solving is self-evident: when you don't even put forth the effort, you can't begin to solve a problem. The tank response doesn't involve failing at your project as much as it does failing to truly show up. Your body might be in the right place—at a meeting or behind your desk—but mentally and emotionally, nobody's home. You may perform tasks that look like work to an outside observer, but your efforts exhibit no true enthusiasm, commitment, or imagination. In reality, you're just going through the motions. When tanking, you work not to dazzle, or even necessarily to succeed; you work merely to get by. Often the problem shifts from how to solve the questions confronting you to how you can most effectively evade them and save face.

Physiologically, people who tank are in a state of low arousal—their heart rate is low, their muscles are slack, their alertness biochemicals are most likely depressed. The "tank posture" includes a lowered head, slumped shoulders, and an expression that suggests defeat. As with athletes, whose fallen face and discouraged disposition can instantly betray a sense of resignation, you can usually recognize the tank response by an idle slouch and air of surrender.

Another sign of the tank response is the constant volley of excuses issuing from the tanker's direction. Continuously rationalizing their record of missed opportunities and justifying their reluctance to act, people who tank never cease pointing out how they were powerless to solve the problem or make their project a success. Some telltale phrases of the tank response: "Who needs that customer?" "That's against our policy." "That department is so hard to work with." The tanker has no shortage of ways to explain away his or her lack of effort and action.

Of all the responses to the challenges of the new working realities, I think tanking is the most insidious, on both a personal and a professional level. In today's business environment, you simply cannot afford to slough off problems. That type of emotional disengagement leads to stale products, neglected customers, and inefficient operations—which lead to ruin. The only way to compete in this world of change and innovation is to devote every ounce of your energy, excitement, and imagination to your tasks. Tanking creates just the opposite behavior: a habit of thinking and action dominated by a sense of listlessness and resignation.

With downsizing, diminished corporate loyalty, and heightened concerns about job security, some degree of emotional withdrawal isn't surprising. But in a wider context, you have to consider the impact of allowing yourself to sink into a mire of cynicism and inaction. Tanking affords no pleasure. Ducking a challenge is totally without savor. Even in ambiguous circumstances, refraining from diving into your problems ends up leading to boredom and stagnation. For many people, the tank response at work extends into life in general—pretty soon, they live their entire life as if they're just trying to get it over with.

THE TENSION RESPONSE—FIGHT OR FLIGHT

"Some people think that when you get serious and intense, things get done," says Glenda Haines, the manager at Public Service of Colorado. "I've never found that. When I look back at times when I'm stressed, I always realize that I didn't do anything constructive. I definitely don't think anyone gets good ideas when they're stressed and tense."

Stress, of course, is a relative phenomenon. Scientifically, the word refers to a heightened state of physiological arousal in response to a perceived threat. In themselves, stressful situations have no definite effect on your ability to solve problems. The fact that you have a big deadline on Friday may provoke an inefficient state of worry, or it may launch you to a new level of exertion and productivity. At a certain point, however, the pattern becomes standard: heightened external pressures lead to an internal feeling of anxiety. If you have two big deadlines on Friday, and both are running behind schedule, then you may very well feel panicked. And the inner state of anxiety that this type of situation creates—what I call the "tension response" to problems—can undermine your ability to think sharply, make good decisions, and effectively interact with other people.

The tension response partially derives from our evolutionary makeup, as a physiological defense mechanism that arouses energy and vigilance in order to fend off danger. In former times, when confronting physical peril, such a surge in alertness and intensity allowed our ancestors to fight off predators—or outrun them if they were particularly large and nasty. But while invaluable in ages past, this defense mechanism is largely inappropriate for today's less physically predatory, more mentally complex world. Unless your organization has developed a new problem-solving protocol that involves Indian wrestling or hundred-yard dashes, this physiological arousal hinders rather than helps your performance.

HARDENING OF THE CATEGORIES

The tension response embodies a spectrum of emotions ranging from full-flushed anger to debilitating fear. But because for most people emotional extremes are rare, I'm going to talk about the two most prevalent reactions within this domain. Getting upset in the face of problems represents one of the most common manifestations of the tension response. In fact, a recent *New York Times* poll revealed that compared to the 8 percent of the working population who think that the office environment is friendlier than it used to be, 53 percent think an angrier mood predominates. You get delegated an unwanted assignment, your budget gets slashed, your team fails to appreciate the genius of your latest idea—some form of injustice strikes, and it pitches you into a state of resentment and frustration. Your shoulders tense up, your jaw tightens, and a scowl affixes itself firmly to your face. While you're in frustration mode, persons crossing your path meet with curt or possibly disparaging treatment. The tasks you undertake receive distracted, shortsighted attention.

So many people automatically respond to problems by getting upset that people think it's an appropriate or even an effective reaction. We've gotten the impression it betrays a manly, John Wayne kind of response—an attitude conveying the idea that we mean business. In truth, getting upset over problems is an excessive, self-indulgent response. It's almost as if the angry person believes that a problem constitutes an affront to what should be a flawless road to success, rather than a step in the process of learning and work.

Anger sometimes serves a purpose. It can allow you to marshal your strength to address a perceived wrong, or prompt you to probe your feelings about an important issue. But far more often, anger or frustration predisposes you to overblown, counterproductive behavior. Psychologically, anger clogs thinking. Like saturated fat produces a hardening of the arteries, anger produces what you could call "hardening of the categories"—an inability to see options that results in stereotyped thought processes. Physiologically, getting upset correlates with an elevated heart rate, tense muscles, and an overly generous supply of "stress" hormones coursing through your body and brain. Generally, you're poised to squander your time and energy, render thoughtless judgments, and cause others to find you repugnant.

HIGH ANXIETY

A second manifestation of the tension response is reacting with worry or anxiety. Problematic tasks, such as attempting to resolve the impediments to a major deal or struggling to adjust to a new restructuring in your department, often provoke nervousness and fear. In fact, the hectic pace and heavy workloads that most people face make a moderate level of worrying a standard state of existence. As we discussed, some degree of anxiousness can propel you to work harder and concentrate more intently. But at a certain point—a point that I believe many people regularly cross—anxiety taxes your mind, dispels your focus, and reduces your ability to perform. At its worst, you could think of this as the "Woody Allen response," based on his frequent roles as a hand-wringing, self-reproaching character who manages to wind himself up into feverish pitches of anxiety.

Jim Haymaker, Vice President at Cargill, is acutely aware of the corrosive influence of anxiety on your ability to think. As head of Cargill's internal consulting department (known as Strategy and Business Development Department), Haymaker acts as an orchestrator of problem solving: "Much of what we do here is structured problem solving and concentrated thought, and that can be hard work." Since his teams are often called in to help various divisions of Cargill with their fundamental strategic problems, the personal pressure can be severe: "In this kind of work—where we are with business units, struggling with them on their toughest problems—you tend to carry problems with you in your head, and you're working on them relentlessly." This is the kind of intensity that can easily lead to anxiety. And especially when you're working on complex intellectual tasks, anxiety can undermine your ability to concentrate, communicate, and give birth to new ideas. "Whenever anxiety hits you," Haymaker says, "it tends to shut down internal systems. People tend to freeze up, they become less tactful, less articulate, and less focused." (Cognizant of the need to keep people at top levels of motivation and vitality, Cargill has implemented a well-designed initiative for reasonable work hours, flexible schedules, and the encouragement of outside interests.)

Like anger, worrying can be useful. To the extent that it focuses your mind on a problem, it serves a valuable function. But the majority of thoughts devoted to worrying and anxiety provide a far less helpful service. On average, anxious thoughts are not nimble creative thoughts, but scattered ones. Instead of initiating fresh paths of thinking or novel approaches of investigation, worrying tends to revolve around potential failures and catastrophes. Chasing themselves around in a downward spiral, these racing worries reinforce feelings of helplessness and dread. Rather than helping to solve the problem, this emotional response usually leaves you acting erratically or stuck in the same rut of thought.

As research demonstrates, these negative moods of anger and anxiety hinder your ability to solve problems. One prominent study on anger, for example, demonstrates that angry people think rigidly and act more vindictively. A compilation of studies investigating the effect of anxiety on academic performance provides convincing evidence of the detrimental relationship between worrying and thinking: 126 studies of more than 36,000 people revealed that the more prone a person is to worry, the worse his academic performance (based on a wide variety of tests and measures). Studies involving air traffic controllers demonstrated similar results. Even if they scored better on intelligence tests, air traffic controllers who consistently responded to the pressure of their jobs with anxiety had a much higher rate of failure in the field.

In addition to the immediate diminishment of performance, the tension response can impair your long-term health, vitality, and energy-producing capabilities. Prolonging the heightened state of physiological arousal associated with anger or anxiety increases your risk of high blood pressure, heart disease, and stroke. In terms of your ability to respond to problems, a continual flood of "stress" hormones can wear down the system that produces this physiological arousal. Just as continually driving at full speed leads to a breakdown of the systems that power your car, constantly evoking states of anger or anxiety wears down the tissues and cells that generate energy and mental alertness. Reaching this stage induces an apathetic, exhausted state commonly known as burnout.

Sometimes the best way to get out of the tank or tension responses is to defeat them on a physiological level. Strategies such as exercise, taking a break, or performing a deep-breathing exercise dissipate anxiety and create a fresh perspective on your situation. But on an emotional level, the process involves awakening yourself to the presence of these negative moods, exposing them for the cowardly gripes they are, and showing them no tolerance. Such action marks the beginning of the shift into the challenge response.

THE CHALLENGE RESPONSE—I LOVE PROBLEMS!

As a senior partner with Deloitte & Touche Consulting Group, Steve Baldwin regards problem solving as his chief obligation. "My job is to solve problems—to ferret them out, to deal with them on a timely basis," Baldwin says. "I look forward to having them—to drawing up a list of problems and going to work on them."

Baldwin's sentiment epitomizes the challenge response to problems. Rather than succumbing to states of anger, nervousness, or resignation in the face of demanding circumstances, responding with a sense of challenge enables you to dive into the struggle with a sense of positive excitement. While embodying all the characteristics of the energy zone—energy, confidence, calmness, flexibility, focus, and fun—the challenge response concentrates them on the problem at hand. Rising above the elements that inspire frustration or worry, people in the challenge mentality focus on the opportunities for learning new information and skills, the chance for accomplishing a tough assignment, and the potential for engaging in an exhilarating experience. More than making a stressful situation more tolerable, mastering the challenge response affords you joy in attacking difficulties. You don't just deal with your problems; you sniff out new ones, hunt them down, and relish the process of coming up with astonishingly great solutions.

Adopting the challenge response to difficult circumstances creates a new situation. As in quantum physics, which describes how the nature of light depends on the way it is observed, the very nature of the problem changes when viewed from the challenge mentality. What was once distressing and insurmountable is now manageable, exciting, and maybe even outright fun. What before was sterile is now charged with possibility.

Reframing the Problem

The key to adopting the challenge response when facing a daunting task is to reframe the problem. Reframing a difficult assignment opens the door to a sense of enthusiasm and confidence by defrocking it of its intimidation and putting it in perspective. I often use the metaphor of going from a close-up to a long shot in cinematography to explain this phenomenon. A close-up shot places a tight, narrow frame around a scene, often engrossing the viewer in a single face, object, or action. When you pull back or "reframe" the scene, however, the viewer immediately glimpses the wider, more comprehensive perspective. The subject matter that initially overwhelmed your perceptions becomes only a small part of a much larger picture. This act of viewing the object in a wider context allows you to engage it with a new sense of interest, meaning, and control.

I'm sure you've experienced an equivalent situation at work. You're so overwhelmingly focused on your pet project, for instance, that you lose sight of the bigger picture. For Kimberly McNally, Manager of Education Services at Valley Medical Center outside of Seattle, creating a sense of perspective means interpreting a situation from a long-term view: "I always ask myself

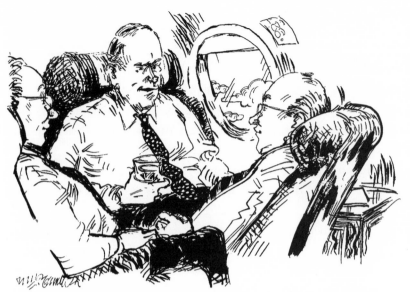

"Sure I like riding the booms—but what I love is defying the slumps."

how important this problem will be one month from now or one year from now." Preoccupation with a particular problem often activates anxiety and myopia, and predisposes you to the tension response. But by putting the problem in context—seeing it as a relatively minor episode in the overall drama of life—you release yourself from many of its worries and open yourself to new possibilities. Such perspective-shifting actions are the initial steps toward converting anxiety into a sense of challenge.

You can also reframe a problem by comparing it to other situations in your life. Remembering other trials or adversity you've come through can help you realize that you're capable of handling difficult situations. Pat O'Donnell, the CEO of Aspen Skiing Company, often attributes his ability to stay calm and focused in a tough meeting to his rock-climbing experiences many years ago. "When things are really frenetic," O'Donnell says, "I think back to being out on the face of El Capitán about 2,000 feet up when my feet were slipping on a piece of glasslike rock. You have to stay there and relax until you get yourself under control." Thinking of the incident makes any deal he's in—even crucial ones—not seem too formidable. "I sometimes equate that event to my day-to-day activities here. Somehow that puts everything in perspective and keeps me going mentally."

A final critical component to reframing a difficult problem as a challenge involves consciously considering the ways it will contribute, in the long run, to your skills and personal development. Keeping an eye toward the ways that a trying experience will improve your expertise and abilities remains one of the most valuable ways to inject a spirit of meaning, determination, and excitement into your work. It helps, in particular, to realize that the tougher the assignment, the steeper the learning curve, and the more dramatic the change, the more knowledgeable, confident, and competent you will emerge. In fact, as Morgan McCall Jr., Michael Lombardo, and Ann Morrison show in their book *The Lessons of Experience*, people overwhelmingly report that there is no better teacher than a difficult problem. In the hundreds of interviews the authors conducted with executives around the world, not one person reported a significant expansion of competence, advancement in knowledge, or personal growth during routine, predictable, static situations. On the other hand, they pointed almost invariably to their toughest, most challenging assignments (being sent to a foreign country to establish a branch or being designated to design and market a totally new product) as their most valuable—and most exciting—experiences. In other words, if you are currently entangled in an arduous problem, then you are involved in a significant, challenging, and memorable experience. Use this realization to engage the struggle with fitting boldness and delight.

Apart from reframing strategies to put problems in perspective, adopting the challenge response means awakening yourself to the exhilaration of engaging in a challenging task. As Sherlock Holmes thoroughly enjoyed stalking clues, assembling the pieces, and cracking the case, you have to learn to relish the problems that accompany the process of building a great product or designing a brilliant business strategy. Far too often we flee from hardship, thinking of its toil and conflict. But to adopt the challenge mentality, you have to learn to love embroiling yourself in intense situations and take pleasure in the chance to test your stamina and skill. While different from the enjoyment of a beach party, most problems have great and underexploited potential to be sources of excitement and fun.

One of the most vivid demonstrations of becoming challenged in the face of adversity comes from the four officers who are at the helm of VisionTek, one of the nation's leading memory-chip manufacturers. I first learned of the Gurnee, Illinois-based VisionTek when reading the *Inc. 500* list of the nation's leading small businesses (the company had 1995 revenues of $450 million) and was intrigued by stories of their upbeat office environment and emphasis on fun. (VisionTek's office facility, for example, includes a spacious indoor basketball court on which employees regularly converge to do their Chicago Bulls impression.) Interested in meeting the officers and scoping out the environment, I set up an interview.

Just before getting on the plane to visit them, however, I came across a second article on the company, this one decidedly less whimsical. A precipitous 75 percent drop in memory-chip prices had recently blindsided the industry; VisionTek's 1996 revenue was forecasted to decrease by half. Thinking the atmosphere might have taken a similar downturn, I wondered whether I should even make the trip. But my doubts were unfounded: it turned out that the level of emotional energy seemed sharply up.

"Now that business is tough, I've never been more into it," Allen Sutker, the Chairman and President, told me. Attired in shorts, black Nike high-tops, a casual short-sleeved shirt, and a gold earring, the 35-year-old Sutker's definition of "being into it" is a little different from that of most people. But unquestionably, Sutker is fully engaged in VisionTek's challenge—not just exhibiting resilience under pressure but rallying the entire company at this improbable time to new levels of excitement and enthusiasm. The co-owners with Sutker—CEO Mark Polinsky, CFO Craig Gutmann, and Vice President Scott Dauer, good friends of Sutker's from childhood—have reacted to the onset of adversity with similar optimism and determination. Diversifying into new products, laying out a new strategic focus, and reinforcing their sales efforts, the company has elevated their activity along with their attitude. As Sutker says, "It really woke us up. Before, a monkey could have made money in memory—it's now that it's a challenge that I'm pumped up." Polinsky's mentality betrays the same spirit: "Anyone can do well when things are going well. When things are tough, that's when you find out how good you really are."

By nature, Sutker is a very competitive person ("I hate losing with a passion"). But one of his strengths—and a key element to transforming a difficult problem into a challenge—is his ability to approach the situation like a game. Despite the recent downturn, Sutker says, "I have the ability to remove the pressure from myself and really focus on the challenge that's at hand. It's one big game. Every problem is part of the game." And as the entire of-fice environment attests, he invests the game with a contagious level of confidence, enthusiasm, and fun. As Sutker says, "We're really excited. We know we're going to win."

As I expected, the VisionTek group was busy—I had received a call before our meeting saying that our interview time was lim-ited. I assumed the officers would be racing between budget meetings and strategy sessions. But it turned out that they had a crucial golf game that afternoon. "We realize we gotta get good at golf," Sutker said of himself and one of his teammates, who are newcomers to the game. "If we can get good on the golf course, then we'll be really deadly."

Like the tank or tension response, the challenge response cor-responds to measurable changes in your physiology. Responding to problems or pressures with an attitude of enthusiasm, humor, and challenge leads to a state of heightened physiological arousal characterized by high energy and mental alertness. As with the tension response, you have an elevated heart rate, higher blood pressure, and more blood glucose available for energy utilization. But unlike the tension response, the challenge response is associ-ated with only a slight rise in heart rate and blood pressure. In other physiological measures, the moods produce very different changes: whereas anger or anxiety stimulates tense muscles and shallow breathing, a confident, enthusiastic attitude corresponds with loose muscles and deep breathing. Biochemically, both the tension and challenge responses induce the secretion of epinephrine and norepinephrine. But again, while worry and tension promote excessive levels of these biochemicals—plus the secretion of cortisol, a hormone associated with negative stress—a challenge mentality produces them on slightly raised and balanced levels with little or no cortisol. In general, these physiological changes help create the state of body and mind in which you think at your clearest, work with enthusiasm, and solve problems most effectively.

These physiological effects of the challenge response also exert tremendous influence on your long-term physical health and vitality. In fact, a number of studies show that an attitude of challenge and determination is one of the best predictors of your rate of illness (the stronger the challenge attitude, the lower the rate of illness). Other research indicates that, among people who work long hours, the key difference between those who feel worn out and discontent and those who feel confident and satisfied is their attitude—people who work with a positive sense of energy used the stress to propel them to higher levels of performance and self-mastery. The scientific verdict is clear: the challenge response prepares you in both the short and the long term for higher levels of exuberance and superior capacities for problem solving.

Rising to the Challenge

"The whole of life lies in the word *seeing*," said the famous paleontologist and philosopher Teilhard de Chardin. Seeing a tough situation from the challenge response instead of the tank or tension response completely alters its shape and meaning. It opens you up to the opportunities for learning and excitement, and creates a state of body and mind in which you think and function optimally. With the tremendous changes and responsibilities of today's world, there is no other answer but to master your response to problems, to pride yourself on being a great problem solver, and to learn to love the process.

CATCHFIRE TIPS FOR LEARNING TO LOVE PROBLEMS

1. *Realize that a changing world spews forth problems.* Solving problems isn't a personal imposition; it's your job.
2. *Reframe the problem.* See your problem as a puzzle or game. Discover its hidden sources of fun. Take advantage of the opportunity to learn.
3. *Distinguish between solvable problems and unresolvable predicaments.* If it's a problem, get down to work; if it's a predicament, realize you have to create new ways to cope with the situation.
4. *There is no problem so big you can't run away from it.* Leave the office, do some exercise, and return to the problem fearless and sharp.
5. *Recognize the symptoms of the tank response.* Straighten up, stop complaining, and force yourself into challenge mode.
6. *Pay attention to your tendency to get nervous or angry.* Step back from the problem, take a deep breath, and tackle it with excitement, not exasperation.
7. *Repeat 25 times a day "I love problems."*

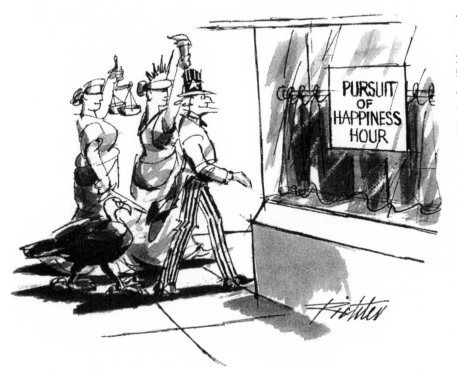

Putting Humor to Work: The Director of Mirth

I love humor as an interlude not to take the focus off the problem, but to recognize the reality of the situation. Humor is about an acknowledgment that, as a human race, we're probably pretty funny to look at.
—Thomas Tierney, CEO, Body Wise International

A t the base of the buildings of Mutual Life of Canada in Waterloo, Ontario, sits the Garden Court, a lovely courtyard with a tasteful fountain and a pleasant little waterfall. On any given day, a stream of professionally attired men and women bustle through the area to and from their meetings and appointments. But one day last summer, as people made their way through the courtyard, something stopped them short.

A diver—clad from head to toe in wet suit, flippers, and mask—was doing the backstroke in the fountain. Interrupted from their busy thoughts of financial products and insurance company procedures, many people were prompted by the sight to burst into laughter. Accompanying the laughter was a feeling of amused puzzlement: Who the hell was this lunatic in the company fountain?

That, in fact, was the question asked by a sign posted near the fountain. And if you thought you knew the diver's identity, you were to e-mail the Mirth Committee—the name of the group that concocted this stunt—in hopes of winning dinner at a great Waterloo restaurant. The totally ridiculous spectacle caused a hefty crowd to gather, place bets on the identity of the masked man, and share a round of high-spirited hilarity. (The mystery swimmer, it turns out, was Dan Lauzon, Director of Sales Force Compensation, who reportedly cuts a mean figure in a wet suit.)

The man-in-the-fountain caper is one of many humorous episodes that regularly surface in the Individual Division of Mutual Life. The department, fearlessly led by a self-organized Mirth Committee, has become famous for its efforts to make work interesting, enjoyable, and sometimes even hilarious. And management doesn't just tolerate it—they encourage it. In fact, they've made it official. When the division presented its 1996 Business Plan, one of the six key objectives outlined for the $200 million yearly budget—along with such initiatives as expanding the sales force and creating new financial products—was to build more mirth into day-to-day activities.

Mirth? Some managers in the company were skeptical. But despite the nature of the subject, Executive Vice President Barry Triller and the rest of the division were serious. Although Mutual Life was thriving (they had just sold $1 billion of insurance in a month—the first time a Canadian company has ever reached that milestone), more competitors were entering the market and more changes in the industry were brewing. In order to maintain top performance in the face of such pressures, people needed the enthusiasm, laughter, spontaneity, cheerfulness, vigor, and flexibility that a sense of mirth affords.

I've heard many people—managers especially—talk about how "it's good to have fun at work every now and then," only to see them acting in ways that suffocate a humorful spirit. But from my work with Triller and Mutual Life, I know that he actively cultivates a positive sense of humor himself, and joins with others to promote it throughout the entire division. Not long ago, when I was in Waterloo to speak at Mutual's annual kickoff meeting, Triller addressed hundreds of people from his department about the outlook and goals for the upcoming year. Even as he discussed the tough new demands of the strategy, the bright, multicolored fool's cap perched atop his head and the absurdly oversized yellow glasses engulfing his face staunchly proclaimed that this was a man who was serious about his mirth.

Corporate Anhedonia— Being Humor-Impaired

Exhibiting a sense of humor at work violates what many people consider businesslike demeanor. Cracking jokes and fooling around, according to this line of thinking, distract your focus from work and undermine the seriousness of your tasks. If not outright subversive, these actions decrease efficiency and promote intolerable attitudes of silliness and frivolity.

Of course, freewheeling frivolity, as in excessive clownishness or unmitigated hedonism, can reduce your productivity and disrupt the people around you. But what seems to me far more damaging to most corporate environments is a different kind of frivolity—the frivolity of being overly serious. In other words, rather than suffering from an outbreak of silliness, it is much more common for companies to be waylaid with what psychologists call *anhedonia*—the inability to experience pleasure and fun. This malaise partially stems from an industrial age mind-set, an attitude of grimness and drudgery that recalls a gruff factory foreman from a century ago. It also comes from contemporary conditions of hectic schedules and demanding workloads. But whatever the source, many people are not enjoying themselves on the job. As Steve Baldwin, whose work as a senior partner of Deloitte & Touche Consulting Group has exposed him to numerous corporations, says: "Do many companies come with a sense of humor? No. There's a lot of insecurity, and there's a reluctance to let down your guard and introduce humor into the situation."

The point is that a prevailing mentality of sternness and sobriety is not only boring, it constitutes a significant business liability. When seriousness reigns unchecked, people tend to grow uptight and rigid. Their thinking becomes sluggish and dry. Their meetings, phone messages, and letters are characterized by an excruciating blandness. Nothing about their presence stirs the soul. In terms of interpersonal skills, the common stodginess and self-importance of the overly serious can ruin their chance to build open, congenial, profitable relationships. As Baldwin says, "It's really an impediment to communication and enjoyment." Put simply, mental and emotional drabness cripple your capacity to create outstanding products and companies.

The worst part is that many people don't realize that they're not having fun. Totally immersed in their work, they fall into the belief that plowing away in a state of cheerlessness and apathy is an acceptable mode of existence. Only in rare moments of lucidity do they discover that they've lost their sense of zest and joy, and recognize that their work—not to mention their life—shows it.

Are You Having Fun Yet?

I've conducted an informal study of humor since my master's thesis on humor in the works of Mark Twain. Along the way, I gained a keen appreciation of the power of humor to move people, whether it be to disarm, incite, or enlighten them. When I began to investigate the mind-body aspects of human performance, this understanding of comedy led me to read with interest about the scientific effects of humor on attitude and coping style, as well as its tangible impact on biology. Interviews with such humor experts as Norman Cousins and Dr. Steven Forness of UCLA and Dr. Harvey Mindess of Antioch College reinforced my long-standing belief that a sense of humor is a hallmark of health, vitality, and ingenuity. (And lest it be thought that I approached humor solely through the dry pages of journals and books, I have always made a point to attend festive gatherings, generously spread jokes, and drink healthy amounts of wine—all in self-sacrificing devotion to science and scholarship.)

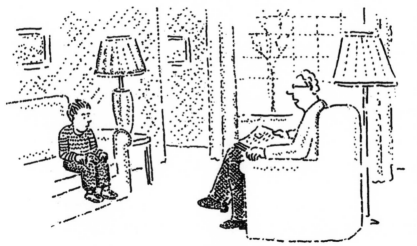

"Go out and play, Norman—it's your job."

Humor, of course, encompasses a great variety of shapes, subjects, and styles. It finds expression in jokes, impressions, cartoons, movies, literature, and stand-up comedy, to name only a few. Its tone ranges from innocent and good-natured to high-spirited and hilarious to critical and cruel—and even to other dimensions of eccentricity and weirdness. But what I mean by a sense of humor is humor in its best sense—a positive, lively, mirthful spirit, a state of fun, an attitude that sees the lightheartedness and comic twists even in difficult situations. Of course, I heartily encourage putting yourself in the way of people and events that provoke uncontrollable convulsions of loud laughter. But the point isn't to get you dressing up in wet suits or streaking through the office, if that's not your style. The underlying force of humor—the shift in attitude that puts you in a high-performance state of mind—comes from a certain Zen-like ability to appreciate the absurdity of life and then to jump in anyway, seizing as much joy and excitement as possible.

Cultivating this type of humor—Step 6 of the CatchFire program—engenders the mental and emotional state in which you perform optimally. From a physical point of view, laughter and a state of fun stimulate many of the same positive physiological changes as exercise: deeper breathing, lower heart rate, decreased blood pressure, and a general feeling of relaxation. On an emotional level, being in a state of fun enables you to enliven situations with amusement, build relationships, and resist the snare of entangling yourself in your work with excessive preoccupation. Mentally, a humorful mind-set bestows a sense of perspective and (as many studies have shown) spurs more expansive thinking and creative problem solving. Overall, humor engenders a powerful, even somewhat miraculous sense of balance, perspective, and joy that allows you to flourish in the midst of a tough business environment.

The vast majority of the respondents of the Professional Workforce Survey agreed: a towering 90 percent said that humor helps them perform better on the job. The differences between people who said they had a good sense of humor and those who didn't were dramatic: compared to the humor-impaired, the mirthful lot were twice as good at sidestepping frustration, eluding anxiety, and pulling themselves out of a bad mood. Additionally, while 50 percent of the humorful crowd reported top levels of energy, only 17 percent of the humorless said they were among the most energetic. In other questions rating their levels of stress, attitude, and performance, people with a sense of humor consistently report a significant advantage.

A Brief History of Humor

The word *humor* comes from the Greek word for fluid, referring to the four bodily fluids (blood, phlegm, bile, and black bile) they believed circulated through the body. In the Greek conception, the particular combination of the fluids in your body determined your mood, which in turn determined your thinking. When out of kilter, these humors produced states of melancholy, sluggishness, or irritability. When in balance, on the other hand—when you were of good humor—you were healthy, happy, and mentally sharp. (While their schema has its obvious faults, the overall analysis of how physical fluids affect moods and thinking corresponds surprisingly well to what contemporary scientists believe about the functioning of neurotransmitters and hormones in the body and brain.)

Although few civilizations had such a complex alchemical description of humor, virtually all societies accorded the comic spirit a significant place in their customs and culture. Often there existed a specific position or a trickster figure—such as the Greek god Pan, the American Indian character Coyote, or the court jester of European monarchs—who embodied the vital sense of humor and play. While some were more mischievous and disruptive than others, their sacred role was to infuse their community or tribe with a sense of joy, excitement, and wonder.

The court jester or fool of medieval and Renaissance times is my favorite of these figures. Any self-respecting king, queen, or nobleman of these eras employed a fool to bring mirth and merriment to the court and kingdom. It's hard for us to imagine, but fools were commonplace figures in the households of any family of stature, and their abilities to entertain were a matter of pride and prestige to the family name (a good fool was roughly equivalent to a top-of-the-line Mercedes). Whether at a feast or in the midst of a difficult ordeal, the antics and acrobatics, witticisms and whimsy, outrageous language and outlandish ploys of the fool would provoke the court's laughter at their situation and at themselves. In addition to amusement, the court jester furnished his audience with new perspectives and unconventional styles of thinking. Not only was the "fool" quick-witted, his challenging viewpoints provided wisdom and proportion to the king's thinking as well.

Unfortunately, we've lost much of this spirit—the exuberance and play as well as the balance and perspective—at precisely the wrong time. In today's world of challenge and change, the advantages that a sense of humor confers have never been more valuable.

The Physiology of Mirth

At the most tangible level, humor, laughter, and fun have a significant effect on many of the systems of the body. While almost everyone has experienced the way humor can transform your mood or the mood of an entire group, most people don't realize that laughter and a humorful state of mind change the very chemicals and cells of their being. Although far from complete, the research in many areas is extremely persuasive. Not only does a comic perspective mobilize the defenses of your immune system, but it also alters your body and brain in ways that can substantially enhance your mood, your thinking, and your ability to perform at work. When you're having fun, you are physiologically primed to thrive on whatever project or problem crosses your path.

Norman Cousins was the first person to call attention to scientific evidence of the effects of humor on physical health. As chronicled in his books *The Anatomy of an Illness as Perceived by the Patient* and *Head First: The Biology of Hope*, Cousins helped heal himself from debilitating illness—first, a case of collagen disease and later a serious heart attack—by augmenting his treatment with a strict regimen of mirth and laughter (a prescription administered by viewing his favorite comedy videos). Along with other pioneering investigators, Cousins opened up a new field of research that turned from studying what makes people sick to studying what makes them stay vital and healthy. If anxiety and what we perceive as negative mental states can hurt our physical health, then why can't humor, joy, and other positive states enhance our well-being?

Studies show that, in fact, they do. A humorful attitude creates conditions in the body and brain that predispose you to feel relaxed, think expansively, and enjoy whatever task you happen to be undertaking. Laughter, in particular, acts like physical exercise, temporarily producing a heightened state of physiological arousal, and afterward leaving you in a loose, pleasant state. Similar to a brief, very low-impact aerobic session, a convulsive guffaw accelerates breathing, increases heart rate, and elevates blood pressure. For the laugh's duration, the internal systems of your body undergo a healthy surge of activity, one benefit of which is the increased availability of oxygen in the bloodstream and in the brain (a condition that leads to keener thinking). Finally, at laugh's end, physiological factors swing in the opposite direction and leave you in a state of calmness: heart rate and blood pressure are low, breathing is slower and deeper, and the musculature of the body is totally relaxed.

Laughter and play also trigger changes in biochemistry that lead to enhanced feelings of calmness and energy, which, in turn, lead to an improved ability to work. Dr. Lee Berk and Dr. Stanley Tan, research scientists at Loma Linda University in southern California, are two of the leading authorities on this topic. In one of their experiments, Berk and Tan sat a number of people—complete with a maze of IV tubes and assorted wires connecting them to computers and machinery at the sides of their chairs—in front of a large-screened monitor featuring the Marx Brothers. While the wired-up patients responded with great laughter and delight to the Marx Brothers' gibes, the medical machinery took measurements of various biochemicals in their system.

The experiment—a study reported in medical journals and media throughout the world—resulted in some fascinating conclusions. Compared to control groups watching nonhumorous videos, the production of natural killer cells (the cells dispatched by the body to attack the cells of disease) in the immune system of the Marx Brothers viewers was significantly higher. Also, laughter and elation were found to suppress levels of cortisol, the hormone associated with feelings of fear, tension, and pressure. What was somewhat surprising was that endorphin levels in the brain, which other studies found to elevate with laughter, increased by only a very modest amount. Whether endorphins play a significant role or not, however, the subjects who watched funny videos underwent biochemical changes that are associated with many positive results: a greater resistance to illness, and, more to the point, a greater sense of energy, calmness, and joy.

Performing in the State of Fun

The physiological evidence makes clear that laughter and fun produce measurable differences in your body and brain. But the goal here in cultivating a sense of humor isn't to elevate levels of natural killer cells. The purpose is to heighten your enthusiasm, double your enjoyment, and improve your ability to handle pressure at work. And despite the ingrained professional bias against it, more and more people are recognizing how critical these aspects of humor are for business. As Gretchen Shine, General Manager of Cox Cable's Roanoke office, says, "When I walk around, I hear these ripples of laughter throughout the company, which to me is so exhilarating because it says, 'There is an informality here, people are having a good time, and they are working hard.'" Shine thinks it's so important that she checks out the humor profile of potential hirees, and looks askance at those who exhibit a laughter deficiency: "One of the things we do when we're interviewing candidates is we ask, 'What is the last thing you laughed about—not a little chortle but a really loud laugh?' Unfortunately, a lot of people look blank. You can tell that they really haven't laughed a lot. We try to avoid them."

Humor affects your state of mind in a number of different ways. Most fundamentally, it puts you in a relaxed, positive, productive mood, a condition sociologist Max Eastman calls the *state of fun*. A remarkable transformation occurs in the state of fun: the projects you tackle and the situations you encounter—even those ostensibly grueling or dull—become events that provoke interest and laughter. The process of this transformation works by means of two shifts of mind. First, a mirthful attitude instills a sense of lightheartedness and detachment that allows you to play with your problems. Second, it imbues you with a spirit of enthusiasm, enjoyment, and zest—an active desire to see what kind of fun you can stir up with whatever tasks or opportunities come your way. The combined effect is a pressure-relieving, enjoyment-enhancing mind-set that allows you to work on a superior level.

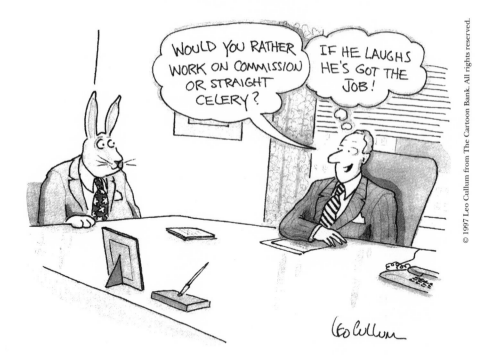

Asobase Kotaba—
Playful Detachment

Mirthful humor creates a sense of lightheartedness, detachment, and play that frees you from rigidity and tension. Levity, in fact, demolishes negative stress, being incompatible with it psychologically and physiologically. When possessed of a sense of detachment, you recognize that worrying won't help solve your problem. You realize that one meeting or project does not encompass the whole of life. As Marty Paradise, General Manager of Microsoft's Southeast District, says, "One thing people have to learn is not to take themselves too seriously." Starting staff meetings by electing a team member to tell a joke, and asking employees and managers "if they are still having fun" at the end of their one-on-one meetings, Paradise works to dispel uptightness and instill a sense of levity. Even in the heat of battle—during a tight negotiation or the last-second efforts to make a deadline—a lighthearted perspective allows you to stay relaxed, find amusement in the situation, and, in the spirit of the fool, use the present material for a good joke.

One of my favorite examples of this sense of play comes from the "play language" used by the Japanese aristocracy many years ago. This play parlance, called *Asobase kotaba*, was a form of speech in which every event is phrased as if you were undertaking it in a spirit of play. Thus, you don't make dinner, you "play at" making dinner; you don't go to Tokyo, you "play at" going to Tokyo. The assumption behind the dialect is that the actor possesses an unassailable spirit of delight, one that leads to an easygoing, isn't-this-amusing mentality. Or as the mythologist Joseph Campbell says, the language contains the marvelous outlook that "the person is in such control of his life and his powers that for him everything is a play, a game. He is able to enter into life as one would enter a game, freely and with ease." It would probably be awkward to adopt this language at work ("I'll play at talking to the client about why they rejected our offer, you guys play at re-creating a brilliant proposal, we'll play at meeting this afternoon, and we can play at having it in the mail by tonight's deadline"). But it makes a critical difference if you can withdraw your worry and apprehensions, stroll onto your stage like an actor or actress, and play your role of account executive, manager of operations, or customer service representative with mastery and delight.

Joyful Relish

In addition to the dispassionate sense of lightheartedness and play, a mirthful attitude helps create a decidedly passionate spirit of excitement and joy. It's a straightforward concept, but one that is routinely ignored: when you expect humor and fun in an assignment, you jump in with greater enthusiasm and perform your tasks with greater delight. Having fun triggers optimism and cheerfulness. As watching a child at play illustrates, it invites total absorption in your activity. Most important, a spirit of mirth elevates levels of energy and exhilaration; your projects become a thrilling sport.

Jim Ruybal's experience managing the Satellite Theatre Network at United Artists aptly illustrates the workings of fun on performance. While the events they broadcast are usually exciting, they compel long hours and intense concentration; sometimes people work from 6 A.M. until 9 P.M. both Saturday and Sunday. What enables them to maintain their spirit during these times, Ruybal says, is "an ability to laugh and have fun." Even if his presence isn't necessary, Ruybal likes to go to the meetings with everyone for the simple reason that the gatherings are a good time, with what he describes as a high school atmosphere. "We have a lot of informal meetings around events—pre-launch meetings, pre-event meetings, post-event meetings—and they're really fun to sit in on. Someone's always there with a quick idea and a funny thing to say. I don't want to say that nothing is sacred, but we kid each other on things that went well and things that didn't go well." While witty exchanges don't need to happen every minute, joking and joviality initiate a higher level of interest, involvement, and even relish of work. Despite what uptight corporate anhedonists say, this spirit of joy drives top performance. As Ruybal says, "If people aren't having fun, they're not giving all they've got. It's impossible to give all your creativity and energies without it."

Creating Relationships

Once his company had taken over a unit of the 3M corporation, Chuck Inman of Alcon Surgical (the ophthalmologic surgery product manufacturer) knew that his team needed to consult with a doctor who had been helping 3M's people. And he knew that the doctor didn't think too highly of the new ownership. As Inman, the Group Product Director, describes it, "we were dealing with someone who thought that Alcon was this big huge company with no personality to it." Hoping that a three-day, face-to-face meeting would break the ice and get things rolling, Inman's group went to visit the doctor and his associates. The beginning stages of the meeting, however, were not just inauspicious, they were terrible: "I took my staff to meet his staff, and the walls just went up immediately. We worked all day long and it only got worse and worse, and the next day the same thing happened."

Though disappointed with the progress and the prospects, Inman took everyone out for a dinner they had scheduled for the second night. At dinner, the relationship finally seemed to inch toward a more agreeable level: "We had a couple of bottles of wine and kind of loosened up, and you could tell that things were changing just a little bit." With this slight encouragement, Inman thought he saw an opportunity to employ a secret weapon. "I looked across at the doctor—a kindly, white-haired gentleman known throughout the world for ophthalmology—and I said, 'That's a beautiful tie you have.' " The doctor was quite pleased with the compliment. This just happened to be his favorite tie, a gift his son had gotten for him in Switzerland. Inman's next comment, however, didn't go over quite as smoothly: "I said, 'I'd like to put a cigarette out on your tie.'

"He looked at me like I was crazy. He said, 'Chuck, I just told you this was my favorite tie. You'd have a better chance of putting an apple on my head and shooting it off with a forty-five.' " But Inman had piqued the group's curiosity, and recognizing his intent to perform a magic trick, they persuaded the doctor to risk the precious neckpiece (in fact, they even provided Inman the cigarette, to ensure he didn't use a trick one). "So I walked over, lit the cigarette, and put it out on the tie," Inman says. "The entire cigarette disappeared, and there was not a trace of anything. Not even a burn mark! They couldn't believe it, and we laughed the rest of the night." (True to the magician's code, Inman wouldn't reveal any details of the sorcery.)

The results of the shared mirth were remarkable. "The next morning they were still laughing and talking about where the cigarette went," Inman says. "And the walls just came down. We got more done that day than the previous two days. The doctor started saying, 'Hey, these guys are all right—it's just a big company made up of normal people.' " From that point on, the partnership flourished. A fun and cooperative relationship had been established, and Inman says they worked together with astonishing productivity:

"You wouldn't believe what we got accomplished. . . . We got more accomplished in the next two months than the previous group had in two and a half years. It was amazing."

While the loose, enthusiastic mood fostered by humor enables you to more effectively tackle your projects and problems, this mirthful state of mind serves another vitally important purpose: it helps you build a good relationship with other people. Humor dissolves barriers and disarms suspicion. Appropriately employed, it promptly rids situations of stiffness and animosity. But even more, laughing, joking, and having fun with someone is possibly the best way to establish a bond with them. As the comedian Victor Borge said, "Humor is the shortest distance between two people." Once you've laughed with someone, you've created an atmosphere of openness, optimism, and excitement that ignites participation and productivity.

In today's age of information, with the prominence of teams and teamwork, it's difficult to exaggerate the importance of this relationship-building quality of humor. If you were merely dispatching or receiving orders, as in a typical industrial age setting, then establishing an environment of openness and interest wouldn't be important. But when your performance and your team's performance depend on your ability to cooperate, share intelligence, and exchange insights, the process is a lot smoother when people communicate in a spirit of generosity and humor. When I see working groups having fun, I see groups that abolish pretension, sidestep pettiness and bickering, think more creatively, and dramatically outperform their humor-impaired counterparts.

And it's not just confined to internal relationships, of course. Humor plays a major role in creating a bond with clients. The rationale remains much the same: if you are pleasant to deal with, if you often have a joke for people, if people look forward to talking with you, then you will create more business. William Merriken, Senior Vice President of Polo Retail Corporation, believes that in the relationship-driven retail business, people with a sense of humor have a tremendous advantage. In fact, he says that people without a humorful attitude rarely make it. "This is such a

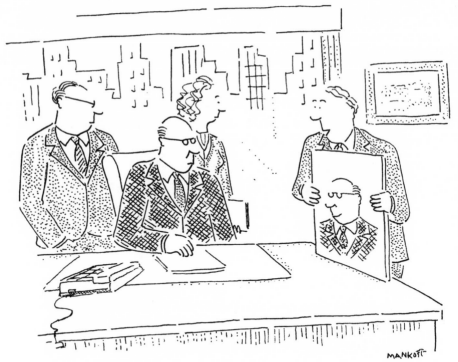

"Here's the artist's conception of your proposed smile."

people business," Merriken says, "you have to have a sense of humor to better interact and make contact with customers. If you don't, you'll self-destruct." As Merriken adds, it's almost part of the job description to show the customer a good time: "Our business is a fun business. People come in because they want to enjoy the experience. They want to be turned on." Marty Paradise of Microsoft wholeheartedly agrees with the sentiment: "Customers want to buy things from people who are having fun and are excited about what they are doing."

To a great extent, every business is a relationship-driven business. Virtually all companies have as a primary goal the cultivation of loyal, long-term customers—the preferred clients who make up the majority of your revenue. With this emphasis on establishing relationships, it's essential to make your interactions personally enjoyable to the people you're dealing with. In a humorful state of mind, such a capacity becomes spontaneous and automatic.

Mind and Mirth

Years ago, a court jester got carried away with his mimicry and mockery of the king. And the king, incensed beyond reason, ordered him immediately put to death. As the guards seized him and started to carry him off, however, a member of the court interceded on the poor fool's behalf. "Good king," the nobleman said, "this fool has served you well for forty years. Surely you will have mercy and change your mind."

Ordering the fool back, the king pronounced a revised verdict: "I'm a divine-right monarch and cannot go back on my word—the fool must die. But because he has been a good fool, I will allow him to choose the *way* he would like to die."

As the court looked on, the fool bowed before the king and said, "If it's all the same to you, sire, I should like to die of old age."

It's no coincidence that fools were known both for their jokes and their quick, inventive thinking: the two are closely intertwined. In fact, research has linked laughter and a mood of elation to more expansive thinking and enhanced problem-solving abilities. By giving our perceptions a good shake, humor opens the door to flexible thinking, creative ideas, and a wider perspective. The fool in the above story offers a perfect example of this. As creativity expert Edward deBono says, "The incidence of humor and creativity are totally interlocked. People that are funny are already creative because they see the improbable and the upside-down logics."

John Cleese, the British comedian who helped create *Monty Python's Flying Circus*, says a sense of humor "gets us from the closed mode to the open mode quicker than anything else." While scientists generally use bigger words in their descriptions, many studies reinforce Cleese's notion. Researchers such as Alice Isen of the University of Maryland, for example, have conducted studies showing that a humorful mood improves your ability to creatively solve problems. In Isen's study, various groups of people watched different videos—one about math, one about exercise, and one that was humorous—and then were asked to solve a problem. While most viewers of the math and exercise videos fell prey to functional fixedness and failed at the task, those who saw the humorous video were often able to devise a creative solution. As Isen says, "The mind associates more broadly when people are feeling good after hearing a joke."

Humor and creative thought are born out of the same mechanism of mind. The punch line of a joke and the "aha" moment of a creative breakthrough spring from a similar source—a shift in perspective, a jump to a different plane, a minor epiphany. The renowned sociologist Arthur Koestler called this mental act the *bisociation of matrices*, meaning the connection of two formerly distinct areas of thought—as in microwaves and cooking to produce the microwave oven. Writers in seventeenth-century England called the capacity "wit"—the combination of seemingly unlike ideas to reveal beauty or genius. Some scientists suggest that this magnificent twist of thought involves greater use of the right side of the brain (the hemisphere associated with images, concepts, and pattern recognition). But whatever its neurological machinations, putting yourself in the state of fun draws out more expansive, imaginative thinking.

Because thinking—and especially innovative thinking—is so critical to business, you should not simply tolerate humor, you should steadfastly enforce it. Functional fixedness and mundane ideas won't get the job done. Being in a humorful mind-set breaks the mold of everyday thinking and launches you to a higher plane of creativity.

Becoming a Resident of the State of Fun

So how do you acquire a sense of humor? The key to developing a better sense of humor, like the key to any change, is awareness. How aware are you of your humor quotient? How awake are you to opportunities to engage in fun? As a pointed refresher, answer the following questions:

- How many times a day do you laugh?
- Are you able to see the humorous side of things on a consistent basis?
- Do your coworkers and friends see you as having a good sense of humor?
- How often do you tell jokes?
- How often do you surprise people?
- Have you brought any fun to meetings you've attended recently?

Having a sense of humor, like most skills, is a "use it or lose it" kind of deal. And many people, unfortunately, seem to have lost it. In times past, the fool could jerk you out of such a state of numbness. But in a typical corporate culture today, it's up to you to initiate a state of fun. The good news is that, if you've realized that you have become slightly too serious or even flat-out dull, you can improve your humor skills. There's not a clear twelve-step program for such a change, but what follows are some fairly simple suggestions that I have found to succeed (often with great fanfare) with many of the companies and people I have worked with. After becoming aware of your current measure of mirth, you have to commit yourself toward developing a sense of humor—a resolution less restrictive than a vow of silence or poverty, but one that can be somewhat tricky to implement. And then you have to practice, as you would practice tennis or the piano.

It's not primarily a matter of perfecting your stand-up comedy routine. Not everyone can be Steven Wright or Bill Cosby. Some people just don't care to play the "humor point position." The essential element is to develop an eye for the humor in situations and a readiness to laugh. Preferably, your mirth regimen will include occasional bouts of uproarious laughter. But for your performance at work, a more relaxed, lighthearted, joyful attitude is what enables you to nullify negative stress, unleash creative thinking, and substantially improve your effectiveness. The first step entails approaching your work—even tough, exasperating situations—with an attitude of humor and play.

ADOPT A HUMOROUS ATTITUDE

Approach your tasks with a determination to make them fun. Sometimes this sounds like an act of self-deception. Are you supposed to try to trick yourself into liking whatever you're doing, even if you actually can't stand it? Well, no, not exactly. If you strongly dislike your work and don't see the possibility of improvement in the near future, then probably the best idea, for you and your employer, is to get out of there as soon as possible.

But to some degree, yes. It's not a matter of tricking yourself, but simply deciding to adopt a different frame of mind. In other words, you can make up your mind that you are going to have fun making your afternoon phone calls, find hidden sources of humor in a boring meeting, or wedge a spirit of joy and adventure into superficially unpleasant circumstances. Like beauty, fun resides predominantly in the eye of the beholder. Or to invoke the words of humor expert Harvey Mindess, "We are capable of adding humor to our repertoire of self-perceptions . . . and in this act, I say, we may exert a greater effect on the course and outcome of our struggles than anyone has yet envisualized." Think of what Robin Williams could do if someone challenged him to have as much fun as possible doing your job.

After going through one of my seminars, an executive at Apple Computer asked me how long it takes to develop a sense of humor. I told him that psychologists such as Robert Ornstein (the author of *Psychology of Consciousness*) suggested that it takes at least twenty-one days of consistent repetition, but that I hadn't actually tracked anyone's mirth development. Saying he found that he had sunk into a state of dullness, he told me he had resolved to become a more humorous and creative leader, as well as a more fun person in general. And he said he'd let me know when it happened.

A few months later at another Apple meeting, he caught up with me and told me that he had, in fact, significantly improved his abilities to create and appreciate mirth. When I asked him about his process, he gave me this account: "Every morning, after I run four miles and take a shower, I turn on my VCR and play one of my favorite scenes from the movie *Beverly Hills Cop.* The clip shows Eddie Murphy shoving a banana up a cop car's exhaust pipe, stalling the cop car and allowing him to get away. It's Murphy at his best—solving a problem with humor, confidence, and bravado. Once I've watched that, my whole demeanor is fun-loving, and I go to work with a loose, exhilarated outlook."

TRAFFICKER IN CARTOONS
Collect and distribute funny cartoons. Even if you don't consider yourself genetically endowed with natural wit, one sure way to encourage your humor habit is to traffic in cartoons. Regularly scan newspapers and magazines for any cartoons that make you laugh—or at least smile. Cut them out and add them to your cartoon file. I find it quite useful to file by category; my own file contains cartoons on subjects such as office, boss, sports (golf has its own subsection), health, relationships, technology, art, and cosmic-bizarre. When I find a business associate or friend who, for instance, takes his golf too seriously, I send him a cartoon about it. Invariably the individual responds, and this rather easy form of humor enhances mutual fun levels and deepens the relationship.

The Mirth Committee of the Printing Industries of America took the cartoon idea a step further and created cartoon boxes in various areas on all five floors of the PIA building in Alexandria, Virginia. Cliff Weiss, the official chronicler of PIA's Mirth Committee, noted that "one notoriously grumpy department tried to deface the cartoons, trashing them and breaking the cartoon box . . . but after a few months of weekly cartoons people genuinely began looking forward to seeing the new cartoons."

The business of cartoon trafficking is vitally important. Cartoons, first of all, should be changed at least weekly, or they become old and stale. Second, they need to be carefully cut and posted, not sloppily ripped or torn. Alan Watts once remarked that "an ill-cooked chicken is a chicken who has died in vain." The same applies to cartoons: render them due importance by displaying them with care.

JUST JOKING

Tell jokes more often. Begin with a strict quota of two new jokes per week. Again, the ability to tell jokes is not as important as the ability to laugh easily and appreciate humor. But frequently telling jokes forces you to find funny material, which in turn forces you to form a network of people who are also on the fun bandwagon. The whole pursuit becomes a self-fulfilling prophecy. Additionally, when you tell more jokes, you dramatically improve your delivery; or in the case of some, you won't improve greatly, but it won't bother you anymore when people (the dullards) don't laugh. Think of it as a chance to expand your risk-taking capacity. You can't lose.

ENLIVEN MEETINGS

Create a tone of fun and excitement at meetings. Within the Native American cultures of the Hopi, Zuni, and Cree, the medicine men played what seems a curious role: they were humorists. Beyond praying, chanting, and using medicines and herbs, their job description included going into serious tribal meetings and getting the participants to laugh, calm down, and lighten up. The role was considered extremely important for clear decision making in the meeting.

Of course, meeting agendas are important. But even a flawless agenda won't matter if people are angry, aren't paying attention, or simply aren't up to contributing their thoughts and ideas. Starting meetings with jokes, cartoons, short clips of humorous videos, magicians, or other catalyzing material can not only help defuse tension but also add a level of novelty, interest, and wit. Steve Baldwin of Deloitte & Touche Consulting Group told me that they began one of their recent national meetings with a stint at Universal Studios: "We had all these stuffy senior-level consultants riding the *Back to the Future* ride and listening to a band on a back street." And the outcome was tremendous. "People were genuinely laughing and saying it was the best meeting they've ever been to, and working sessions were extremely productive," Baldwin says. "Working relationships were formed during the fun that will last for years."

With electronic communication becoming more and more prominent, face-to-face meetings present a great and in some cases rare opportunity to establish relationships and have some fun. Taking time to create a mirthful environment can vastly improve the results.

THE DIRECTOR OF MIRTH

Another idea that I've seen work with tremendous success is to establish a mirth committee at your office. At the aforementioned Printing Industries of America, Dan Robertson, the Chief Financial Officer, served the first term as Director of Mirth. (I told him I thought a CFO as a Director of Mirth was an oxymoron, but at least I knew I'd get the minutes of his Mirth Committee on time.) With the full support of Ray Roper, the CEO, PIA's Mirth Committee has helped set up an environment of fun that has been going for three years, sponsoring a variety of activities—some surreptitious—that include theme days, funny contests, bogus memos, and outlandish pranks. In addition to the genuine appreciation the people at PIA came to have for it, Roper has seen a more tangible result: "The bottom line is that productivity and creativity are up, absenteeism and turnover are down, and the customer is getting better service."

PRACTICAL MIRTH

Perform creative practical jokes. The Mirth Committee at PIA has a great example of an imaginative, tasteful, and funny practical joke. Citing from the minutes of one of the mirth meetings:

> On July 8, the building manager distributed a routine memo to all staff: "This weekend the vendor who installed the cabling in our building will thoroughly clean all of our telephone lines by injecting compressed air into the cables. To control dust and debris that may emanate from your telephone receivers, all staff members are urged to store their telephones in their wastebaskets or to procure special bags from the productions department before leaving work on Friday, July 10."

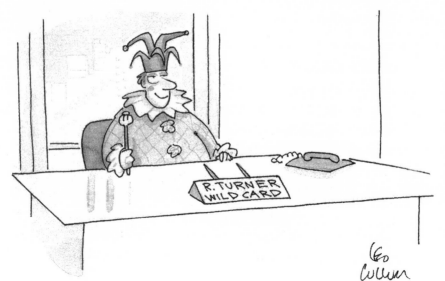

Everyone on staff takes it seriously. The production room is besieged with irritated staff members seeking the special bags. The building manager, who was sworn to secrecy by the Mirth Committee, has no special bags. He improvises an excuse that the bags will be distributed later. By the end of the day, more than half the staff has put in requisitions for the bags. Clear trash can liner bags are actually distributed. One woman who took responsibility for her whole department forgets to procure her bags. She worries all weekend and tries to reach the office manager at home.

The Mirth Committee observes dumbfounded, but no one spills the beans. PIA's president, Ray Roper, who is in on the memo, can be heard laughing uncontrollably in his office in response to a report about the telephone bag activity, but no one suspects.

Over the weekend, members of the Mirth Committee toss sparkly confetti and electrical wire odds and ends into everyone's telephone bag, wrapped secretly around each telephone. That way, no one will feel disappointed. Staff finally gets the message Monday morning: it was just a joke.

Practical jokes heighten excitement and build relationships, which is vital in the new world of information, knowledge transfer, and teamwork.

THE LIMITS OF LAUGHTER

Of course, some forms of humor are inappropriate. And there are times when jokes or pranks will arouse far more resentment than enthusiasm. As I said, I'm talking about humor in the highest sense of the word: fun, joy, and lightheartedness. In fact, the physiological, emotional, and mental benefits of humor discussed here all come from mirthful humor—humor associated with elation and feeling good. Humor deriving from scorn, ridicule, or derision generally has the negative effects associated with feelings of anger or anxiety. Know the people around you, and be sensitive to their concerns.

After relating that, however, I have to say that there aren't too many situations on an ordinary day in the office that are so serious that a skillful flourish of humor would be out of line. Without dismissing the importance and difficulty of your situation, men and women throughout history have laughed in times of war, drought, disease, and poverty. However serious your plight may be, enjoining it with a sense of levity wouldn't represent an unprecedented act of crudeness. As George Bernard Shaw once said about the relationship of humor to something as serious as death: "The world doesn't cease to be funny when someone dies any more than it ceases to be serious when someone laughs."

The Function of Fun

Aside from being an essential ingredient to a happy, well-lived life, humor plays a vital role in top performance on the job. While many people seem to lose their comic nature when they don professional attire and march into the office, the pressure of today's world of work makes a spirit of fun more crucial than ever. Humor creates a state of mind in which you think, handle pressure, and interact with others with greater levels of grace and skill. As Mark Twain wrote in *The Mysterious Stranger*, people have "unquestionably one really effective weapon—laughter. . . . Against the assault of laughter nothing can stand."

CATCHFIRE TIPS FOR PUTTING HUMOR TO WORK

1. *Laugh a minimum of 20 times daily.* If it's been a tough day, catch up before you go to bed.
2. *Adopt a humorous attitude.* What would Robin Williams do to create fun if he were in your place?
3. *Watch at least one funny video or television program per week.*
4. *Start a cartoon file.* Organize it by subject matter and send cartoons out to customers, coworkers, and friends (thereby starting a cartoon chain).
5. *Exchange jokes.* You'll sharpen your delivery and wit.
6. *Humorize your meetings.* Employ funny videos, brief games, cartoons, jokes, hats, or whatever it takes.
7. *Start a mirth committee in your office.*
8. *Realize that life is short.* You'd better start enjoying yourself now. If you really want to have fun, no one can stop you.

> *"Work and play are words used to describe the same thing under different conditions."*
> Mark Twain

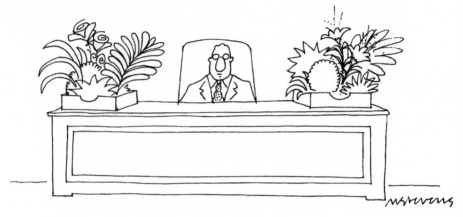

The Greening of Oscar T.

STEP 7

Creating Energizing Environments: From Hindquarters to Headquarters

Environments are not merely passive containers of people but are active processes that reshape people.

—Marshall McLuhan, *The Guttenberg Galaxy*

As sometimes happens, the senior management meeting of the Cadmus Communications Corporation wasn't going well. The debate over important strategy questions had created a tense, unfriendly, and unproductive atmosphere. But luckily, the meeting was in the office building of the division headed by Fredda McDonald (Cadmus Marketing Services), who knew just how to handle the situation. McDonald called time-out and brought in a bunch of big, brightly colored plastic balls to substitute for people's chairs. "I said, 'Hold on—we're taking a break.' I took the chairs out of the meeting room, got the balls, rolled them in the room, and said, 'It's hard to be cantankerous with each other while we're bouncing on these balls.' " As McDonald reports, the balls provided a new, positive environment, and helped everyone calm down and begin a more fruitful discussion. "It totally changed the atmosphere," she says. "We started in with a much better attitude, and had a very productive meeting."

McDonald has designed a work environment at Cadmus Marketing Services that fosters a positive mind-set in a number of different ways, from promoting healthy habits to encouraging a sense of humor. To help employees choose energy-enhancing food, for example, she installed a juice machine and restocked the vending machine with healthy, low-fat snacks. She made an arrangement with a nearby health facility that enables employees to join for a heavily discounted rate, and she encourages them to work out at any time of the day they need a boost. And she imported a gaggle of multicolored balls (exercise therapy balls, actually) that add an element of lightheartedness and joy to the atmosphere. "The purpose of the balls is to promote a spirit of fun," McDonald says. "One ball is in the scheduling room, where the decision making and deadline tension can really be great. It has added a sense of humor to the environment that has proven to be very beneficial."

Most of the CatchFire program helps you cultivate a high-energy, productive mind-set from a mental and physical standpoint—your attitude, thinking habits, humor, diet, exercise, and rest. But an outstanding way to help you implement and sustain these new habits of mind and body involves creating a positive office environment. From making the physical layout of your workplace more interesting and enjoyable, to instituting changes that support healthy eating, exercise, and relaxation, to incorporating items that inject a spirit of fun into your office, you can transform your surroundings into a source of energy and optimism. Most people overlook the fact that your office environment significantly influences your work patterns and mind-set. As Tom Peters emphatically puts it, "We grotesquely underestimate the role of physical space in setting organizational tone." But by following Step 7 in the CatchFire program—creating energizing environments—you can construct an office setting that boosts your health, energy, and productivity.

The Power of Context

The idea for creating an energizing environment comes from Gestalt psychology, which explains how differences in background or environment influence perception. Harvard psychologist Ellen Langer, in her book *Mindfulness*, calls this phenomenon the *power of context.* "The way we behave in any situation has a lot to do with the context," Langer says. "We whisper in hospitals and become anxious in police stations, sad in cemeteries, docile in schools, and jovial at parties. Contexts control our behavior, and our mind-sets determine how we interpret each context."

Unfortunately, most office environments promote lukewarm enthusiasm and bland thinking. Physically, many workplaces are dull and drab. They usually contain some variation of cubicles and small square offices. Meeting and training rooms—where vital company knowledge is imparted, innovative plans are devised, and critical decisions are made—are little better, often consisting of a larger room with a table and chairs. Straight lines, hard edges, and uncomfortable furniture predominate. A sense of professionalism compels many to keep the place impersonal and uninviting.

Most workplaces sap energy in other ways as well. By directly or indirectly supporting poor eating habits, a sedentary work life, and long days of nonstop work, many office environments detract from the health and vitality of their inhabitants. Will Lewis, a consultant and former manager at General Electric, calls these typical boring workplaces *hindquarters* (a place where you rest your butt) instead of *headquarters* (a place that arouses the imagination).

Adroitly redesigning your workspace, however, redirects the power of context to your advantage. The goal is to construct an office environment that pitches you into the energy zone—to make your workplace so inspiring that even if you're lethargic or angry, stepping inside your office and sitting down at your desk transforms you to a high-energy, productive mood. One person who has created such an atmosphere is John Dahlin, President of the advertising agency Dahlin Smith White. "We have to have an environment that's a little loose if we're going to foster creativity and new ideas," says Dahlin in a *Journal of Business Strategy* article. "The physical environment—our office space—was designed to encourage that. None of the walls are straight; they tilt or angle in. There are two or three different door sizes and different windows." Aside from the lively structural design, the agency provides each employee with an art budget to decorate his office (which results in Indian tapestries, sculpted glass heads, and gigantic lightbulbs), and sports a billiards room in the building as well. How does this kind of surrounding affect the people there? "By the time I hit my desk, I'm already jazzed," Dahlin says.

The Hibbert Group, a comprehensive marketing services company with offices in Trenton and Denver, is another example of a company that has created an energizing environment. In conjunction with CatchFire training seminars I conduct at Hibbert with consultant David Pemberton, a committee of employees has redesigned the environment to improve the levels of health, vitality, and humor. "The objective is to create a great place to work," says Bill Walsh, President of Hibbert in Denver and champion of the initiative. "We want to help people do the best work they can for our customers and shareholders. And we think a critical part of working at your best—especially when you're facing a great deal of pressure from tight deadlines and rapid growth—is staying healthy and having fun." To start the redesign process, we worked with the committee to perform an "energy audit" of the facilities, examining the lighting, decor, bulletin boards, cafeteria, vending machines, and overall ambience in the building. Based on the findings, we decided on priorities, sought management approval and funding when necessary, and acted on the decisions.

A couple of the general changes to improve the environment involve the construction of a creativity room and the introduction of a lively daily broadcast over Hibbert's P.A. system. The creativity room—transformed from a plain-vanilla meeting room—contains colorful artwork, exercise balls, and materials such as markers, crayons, flip charts, and white boards to help people hatch great ideas. People hold meetings there when they want innovative thinking or a fun environment. The daily broadcasts, which Walsh calls Radio-free Hibbert, consist of daily announcements such as recent company achievements or employee birthdays, a motivational or philosophical quote, and upbeat music.

On the health front, Hibbert has added nutritious choices to their vending machines and posted literature that teaches people about healthy eating habits. To encourage physical activity, the company sponsors health club memberships for employees. Additionally, the committee has installed bike racks for people who want to ride to work, and they've constructed a basketball court at each of their three Denver locations. Lastly, dance lessons are held at the office a couple times a week at lunchtime, providing an ideal opportunity for people to exercise, socialize, and reenergize for an exuberant afternoon of work.

Hibbert has skillfully promoted a humor initiative as well. Framed cartoons adorn walls and common workspaces throughout the company. Social events and practical jokes occur on a regular basis, ranging from traditional outings—such as an annual company trip to a Colorado Rockies baseball game—to surprise deeds of delight. One ordinary Friday, for instance, managers delivered a dose of mirth by stealthily slipping out and returning to the office in outrageous costumes to deliver "mirth boxes" (containing sundry humorous items) to each employee in the company.

"We can feel a significant change taking place at Hibbert," Walsh says of the efforts. "The positive environment we're creating contributes a great deal to our spirit and performance."

Of course, the extent that you can decorate your office depends heavily on your job and your company. Most people don't have any say about what chair they sit in, much less an art budget. If your workspace has to be "client friendly" or if management doesn't give you much leeway, then you won't be able to fully exercise your creative interior design strategies. (I'm fully aware of the depths of small-mindedness some managers have on the issue: one person related to me how he had proudly tacked on his wall a picture of the baseball team he coached, only to be told the next day to remove it or be fired.)

Nevertheless, almost everyone has some control over his own workspace. Even if you can't implement all the suggestions of Step 7, you can probably incorporate some scaled-down version of them. At minimum, you can design your desk or work area and upgrade your on-the-job health habits to support your personal energy, motivation, and fun. At maximum, you can skillfully lobby your managers, coworkers, and assistants to transform your office into a hotbed of excitement and creativity.

Do-It-Yourself Feng Shui

The first step to creating an energizing environment is to make sure your office allows you to work comfortably and productively. This means taking a fresh look at the basics—your desk, chair, files, bookcases, computer, phone, music, and lighting in your workspace—and making sure the arrangement allows you to work as pleasantly and effectively as possible. In other words, perform do-it-yourself *feng shui*.

Feng shui is a system of colors, symbols, spacing, mirrors, light, and sound believed by the Chinese to evoke certain reactions and vibrations within us. *Feng shui* practitioners say that correct orchestration of these elements promotes *chi*, or energy flow. Many businesses have hired *feng shui* consultants to help with the interior design of their buildings—and most find their suggestions make the environment considerably more pleasant. But better yet, use your own sense of what new arrangements, artwork, or other changes would improve your office. If you're at liberty to rearrange desks and furniture, take a half-day with your team to design an interesting, comfortable, productivity-inspiring environment.

Your own domain—whether it's a cubicle or a corner office—should reflect your values and goals. Choose the pictures, photographs, calendars, flowers, cartoons, inspirational quotes, plants, Nerf balls, and other knickknacks that make your space comfortable and enjoyable. If music helps you work well—and your office environment permits it—keep your favorite focus-inspiring music on hand. (Baroque music such as Bach, Vivaldi, or certain kinds of upbeat jazz entrains your brain waves to high alpha frequency, which is associated with mental alertness and creativity.) Depending on your tasks, playing music you enjoy can help you work more productively.

Just as a coach sets up the locker room with posters, pictures, articles, and motivational quotes to keep his or her team focused on its goal, reorchestrate your environment—from your desk, walls, and computer, to the kitchen, rest areas, and meeting rooms (if applicable)—to design an exciting workplace.

One final suggestion for creating an interesting environment: periodically change it up. Rearranging the office renews perspective and vitality. Even with the same furniture and space, you can create a refreshing new atmosphere by shuffling the design of your workplace. I learned this long ago when my mother used to periodically reorganize our house. I'd get home from school one day to find the living room interchanged with the dining room, and my bedroom swapped with one of my sister's rooms. Though slightly confusing if you were returning late at night to a dark house, the rearrangements never failed to breathe a sense of newness and surprise into a familiar environment.

Promoting Healthy Habits

The second strategy to create a high-energy office environment is to encourage habits that thwart negative tension and promote top levels of physical health and energy. By reframing your office to support healthy eating and relaxation, you create the biochemistry that drives top performance.

If you manage the office, start by adding equipment such as a refrigerator, microwave, and kitchen (if you don't already have them). If you aren't in charge and your office lacks these amenities, start with tactful suggestions about how such items would improve health, energy, and morale. Place a fruit bowl in a central location and trade off filling it with a variety of apples, oranges, bananas, and other fruits. Bring chemical-free popcorn

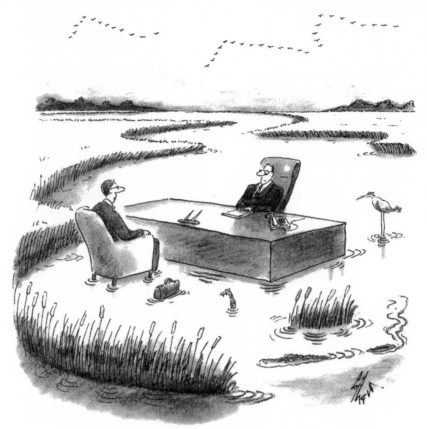

"This isn't your usual habitat."

or high-protein, low-fat energy bars to work. Keep vegetables in your office kitchen refrigerator (most grocery stores carry precut packages of carrots and celery that are a perfect snack). See if you can add healthy, low-fat, low-sugar choices to the vending machines in your office, and check on the possibility of installing water coolers in convenient places. (The vast majority of vending machines that I've checked are stocked with goods that are 90 percent fat and sugar.) Finally, get your company to post health literature in the kitchen and eating areas that informs people about nutrition.

Making changes in your environment is particularly important for your eating habits. When you're hungry or stressed out, or a combination of the two, you'll eat whatever is around. If you stock your office area with fruit and healthy snacks instead of candy and Cokes, you can create physical health and energy rather than exacerbate tension and lethargy.

If possible, designate a comfortable rest area where you can take breaks. Many people find that it's most convenient to close their eyes at their desk for 10 minutes or so for their interval of downtime. But to totally separate yourself from the hustle and bustle of your working environment, having a quiet, relaxing area in which to do some deep breathing or contemplate a problem can work wonders in fighting off fatigue and restoring a sense of calmness. As the mythologist Joseph Campbell says, "To have a sacred place . . . a place of creative incubation . . . is an absolute necessity for anybody today. You must have a room, or a certain hour or so a day, where . . . you can simply experience what you are and what you might be."

Scott Thayer, one of the top-producing consultants at Smith Barney, has created an ideal space for relaxation in his Santa Rosa office. I met Thayer after asking Steve Gesing, the Director of Smith Barney's Consulting Group University, to introduce me to some of the leaders who had energy and passion. When we began discussing office design, Thayer said he insists on creating an exceptional workspace to support exceptional work. When I went to visit him in Santa Rosa, I saw what he meant. In addition to a beautifully designed work environment—complete with full kitchen, impressive technology display, and a terrific art deco fruit bowl placed on an ornate Roman pillar in the middle of the office—Thayer has a deck that he's made into a haven of serenity. The deck has artful ceramic pots, Japanese maple trees, flowers, and comfortable sundeck furniture. And it yields a terrific view of the mountains. "It's a great place to take a break," Thayer says. "If you want to go quiet yourself, you can grab a cup of tea or a banana and go out there and sit in a terrific environment." Other companies such as Xerox and Eastman Kodak have similarly designated rooms for relaxation and fun. In addition to comfortable furniture, these areas are stocked with audio- and videotapes about relaxation exercises, meditation, and humor, and various art supplies to draw, paint, or sculpt your way to a calm state of mind or a creative solution to your problem.

For most people, obviously, such places sound distant from their working world. But creating a scaled-down version of these relaxation areas can still afford a great opportunity to regain a sense of calmness. By using your imagination, you can find some place around your office—a spot in the cafeteria, an unoccupied meeting room, a sofa, a bench outside, or a table in a nearby coffee shop—that you can designate as your place to relax and revitalize.

Fostering Enthusiasm and Fun

A final strategy in designing your office environment is to make it high-spirited and fun. I talked about a number of ways you can do this in Step 6, but the point bears emphasizing. Creating a humorful workplace helps short-circuit anger and anxiety, and fosters openness and enjoyment.

David Palmer, President of Financial Concepts, an investment company in Knoxville, uses toys to create a humorful environment. Palmer has a box full of toys and gadgets on the conference table where he meets with his clients. Whenever he has new customers who are nervous about choosing their life investment strategies, he'll purposefully leave the room "to get a file or a cup of coffee." Invariably the potential clients will start playing with the toys, and one of them will hit the laugh box—a small contraption that emits a loud, outrageous laugh for 30 seconds. Startled and amused, people try to shut it off, looking for a power switch (there is none) and covering up the gadget. While some people get slightly embarrassed, Palmer says, most can't stop laughing, and the outbreak of humor creates a new spirit for the meeting. The laughter dissolves any feeling of tension, reservation, or defensiveness, and Palmer and the client can begin a conversation in a spirit of openness and good humor.

At Public Service of New Mexico, a group of employees used

cartoons in a unique way to humorize the environment. Figuring that elevators were a great place to energize people's mind-sets and emotions, they made one of the elevators into what they called "cartoon alley"—an elevator covered floor to ceiling with cartoons. Everyone riding the elevator would point out and share their favorites with others who were in the elevator at the same time. If you liked one of the cartoons, you could take it and make copies, but you were honor-bound to replace it by the next day. Did it work? In many cases other elevators would stand empty while people waited for the "cartoon alley" elevator.

Here are other ideas to create a humorful environment. Liberally place (and replace, after they've been up for a while) funny cartoons on various bulletin boards, refrigerators, and computers. Decorate your space with objects that keep the climate amusing, such as a small basketball hoop, a dartboard, laugh boxes, toys, or joke books. And put some humor in writing by adding a humor column to the company newsletter. Organize humorous events or contests at work—from joke competitions to humorous videos at lunchtime—or, like Tom Henderson, plan surprises. During stressful periods of work, Henderson, CEO of the Association of Trial Lawyers of America, occasionally rents a popcorn machine, knowing that the scent automatically lifts people up and creates a positive mood. (You can't smell popcorn and be angry at the same time.) Such environmental changes will constantly remind you not to take yourself too seriously, and will encourage a more open relationship with the clients or coworkers who visit your office.

Setting a Meeting Environment

A number of years ago I collaborated with another consultant to help orchestrate an off-site meeting aimed at helping the PepsiCo brand marketing team generate 500 exciting new ideas in their marketing efforts. Taking the group to a resort in Santa Fe, we designed an environment and set up activities to free their minds from the workaday world and unleash their creativity. We ran them up and down the surrounding hills. We had a Mexican Indian scholar discuss the history of the mountain ranges and the visions of ancient chiefs. And we danced to mariachi music as we drank tequila (with limes, of course, to keep us healthy), all in an effort to cast an environment that would give birth to new thinking and ideas. Only after a day and a half did we start on the generation of novel concepts and plans for the marketing campaigns. Knowing the environment had to erase stale, tunnel-vision thinking, we designed the context to widen perspective, open up new thinking, and spark creativity. And we emerged victorious, with over 500 quality ideas, many of which the team implemented over the next few years in their ongoing marketing crusade.

Gearing Up for the Hunt

Creating energizing environments is a potent way to help implement changes in your habits and control your mind-set. In fact, people have been using the power of context for centuries. The caves at Altamira offer an interesting example. Archaeologists identified these caves in southern Spain as a place used by ancient people for refuge and gathering. The carvings and pictographs on the walls of the cave suggest that ancient tribes also used the cave for some ritualistic purposes. The drawings on the cave walls depict objects of the hunt, such as wild boar, deer, and wolves. Some researchers noticed that the flickering firelight made the images come alive, dancing and moving on the walls. They suggested that our ancestors used the pictures to visualize the animals, become focused on their goal, and gather courage and strength for the hunt.

Making healthy, humorous, inspirational additions to your office environment helps create the mind-set that spurs creativity, enthusiasm, and top performance. To paraphrase Marshall McLuhan, we create our environments, and thereafter they re-create us.

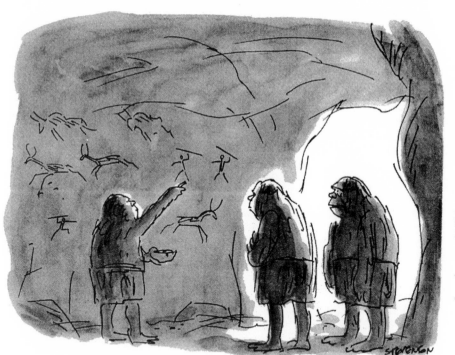

"Someday this cave could be worth plenty."

CATCHFIRE TIPS FOR CREATING AN ENERGIZING ENVIRONMENT

1. *Examine your own environment.* If it's hindquarters, use some creativity to make it a headquarters.
2. *Make the changes.* Take a half day with your team to decide on and implement office design improvements.
3. *Check the lighting of your office.* If it's inadequate, improve it (or lobby management to improve it).
4. *Rearrange your workplace.* Change the arrangement every six months, to a large or small degree.
5. *Make healthful eating easier.* Change vending machines to include more healthy choices, if possible.
6. *Snack on fruit.* Get an office fruit bowl; designate someone in your office to fill it each week.
7. *Create a break room in your office building.* If management won't do it, search out your own relaxation area.

8. *Add fun opportunities.* Build two or three sources of fun into your office, from subtle to outrageous.
9. *Get a therapy ball.* Buy a brightly colored exercise therapy ball for your office.
10. *Rent a popcorn machine.* Or get someone in management to do it.

CONCLUSION
Sparking the Flame

No mariner ever enters upon a more uncharted sea than does the average human being born into the twentieth century. Our ancestors thought they knew their way from birth through all eternity; we are puzzled about the day after to-morrow.

—Walter Lippmann

Working in today's business world means constantly facing pressure and change. Sometimes, meeting the demands of this environment can be difficult; sometimes, it can be overwhelming.

The good news about the fast-paced, high-pressure world is that it forces you to grow and improve your capabilities. Many people are confronting so much change in their job that they become fed up with the continual transformation and forget about the advantages that change confers. Change affords new challenges and opportunities. When I hear the questions of business-people about how to survive change, I often think of the story of the Shushwap Indians of British Columbia, who had an attitude toward change that most people would do well to adopt.

The Shushwap lived on beautiful, plentiful land, with abundant salmon and game. They led peaceful, prosperous, happy

233

lives. Yet the elders of the tribe would periodically call on the people every twenty-five to thirty years to uproot, leave their village and rivers, and find another area to inhabit. Knowing that the lives of the tribe members had grown too predictable, the elders would deliberately force change and challenge: a new village to build, new streams to fish, new hunting trails to establish. While the transition was extremely difficult, it invariably led to the renewal and reinvigoration of the tribe.

As Peter Drucker says, the key to effectively handling pressure or change is to manage your energy. When I met Drucker at a conference in Tarrytown, New York, a few years ago, he said that to be an effective performer "you must first and foremost manage your own energy, and secondly, you must orchestrate the energies of the people around you."

Managing your energy is what the CatchFire program is all about. By putting the seven steps into practice, you gain a sense of vitality and self-control that transforms your life. When you're in control of your energy and emotions, it doesn't matter if you're unsure about what you'll be facing the day after tomorrow. When you've got the energy to face change, the awareness to recognize tough assignments as great opportunities to learn, and the spirit of fun that allows you to embrace the challenges of your career, then whatever problems or crises arise are more grist for the mill. Yes, your work can be taxing. But by practicing the energy-giving steps of the program you can take them on with confidence and gusto, and have fun in situations where no one thought it possible.

To adopt the program, of course, requires dedication and discipline. You have to commit to changes in your attitude and lifestyle that can be difficult to make. Forcing yourself to the health club after a long day of work, wedging a relaxation break into a busy afternoon schedule, or transforming a tense, humorless meeting into an upbeat affair all require a firm commitment to the cause. But while adopting these habits takes time and effort, it returns the expenditure tenfold. The improvements in your energy level, your productivity, and your ability to relish challenges make the commitment an incomparable investment.

BIBLIOGRAPHY

Adams, S. *The Dilbert Principle.* New York: HarperBusiness, 1996.

Bailey, C. *The Fit or Fat Target Diet.* Boston: Houghton Mifflin, 1984.

Bailey, C. *The New Fit or Fat.* Boston: Houghton Mifflin, 1991.

Bailey, C. *Smart Exercise.* Boston: Houghton Mifflin, 1994.

Benson, H., and M. Stark. *Timeless Healing.* New York: Scribner's, 1996.

Benson, H., and E. Stuart. *The Wellness Book.* New York: Simon and Schuster, 1993.

Benson, H. *Your Maximum Mind.* New York: Times Books, 1987.

Borysenko, J. *Minding the Body, Mending the Mind.* New York: Bantam Books, 1987.

Carse, J. *Finite and Infinite Games.* New York: Ballantine Books, 1986.

Chopra, D. *Ageless Body, Timeless Mind.* New York: Harmony Books, 1993.

Chuen, L. K. *Feng Shui Handbook.* New York: Henry Holt, 1996.

Cooper, R. *Health and Fitness Excellence.* Boston: Houghton Mifflin, 1989.

Cousins, N. *Anatomy of an Illness.* New York: Bantam Books, 1979.

Cox, H. *The Feast of Fools.* Cambridge, Mass.: Harvard University Press, 1969.

Csikszentmihalyi, M. *Flow.* New York: HarperPerennial, 1990.

deBono, E. *Lateral Thinking.* New York: Perennial Library, 1970.

Drucker, P. *The Effective Executive.* London, Great Britain: Pan Books, 1967.

Drucker, P. *Managing in a Time of Great Change.* New York: Dutton, 1995.

Edwards, B. *Drawing on the Artist Within.* New York: Simon and Schuster, 1986.

Farson, R. *Management of the Absurd.* New York: Simon and Schuster, 1996.

Freiberg, K., and J. Freiberg. *Nuts!* Austin, Tex.: Bard, 1996.

Gardner, H. *Leading Minds.* New York: Basic Books, 1995.

Garfield, C. *Peak Performers.* New York: Avon Business, 1986.

Glasser, W. *Positive Addiction.* New York: Perennial Library, 1976.

Goleman, D. *Emotional Intelligence.* New York: Bantam Books, 1995.

Grotjahn, M. *Beyond Laughter.* New York: McGraw-Hill, 1957.

Gunaratana, H. *Mindfulness in Plain English.* Boston: Wisdom, 1991.

Gutwirth, S. *You Can Learn to Relax.* Hollywood, Calif.: Wilshire Book, 1957.

Hafen, B., K. Karren, K. Frandsen, and N. Lee Smith. *Mind/Body Health.* Boston: Allyn and Bacon, 1996.

Hammer, M., and J. Champy. *Reengineering the Corporation.* New York: HarperBusiness, 1993.

Handey, J. *Deep Thoughts.* New York: Berkley Books, 1992.

James, W. *The Varieties of Religious Experience.* New York: Penguin Books, 1902.

Kao, J. *Jamming.* New York: HarperBusiness, 1996.

Koestler, A. *The Act of Creation.* New York: Penguin Arkana, 1967.

Kriegel, R., and L. Patler. *If It Ain't Broke . . . Break It!* New York: Warner Books, 1991.

Langer, E. *Mindfulness.* Reading, Mass.: Addison Wesley, 1989.

Larson, G. *The Far Side Gallery.* Kansas City, Kans.: Andrews, McMeel & Parker, 1980.

Leonard, G., and M. Murphy. *The Life We Are Given.* New York: Putnam, 1995.

Loehr, J., and P. McLaughlin. *Mentally Tough.* New York: Evans, 1986.

Maddi, S., and S. Kobasa. *The Hardy Executive.* Homewood, Ill.: Dow Jones-Irwin, 1984.

Maslow, A. *Toward a Psychology of Being.* New York: Van Nostrand Reinhold, 1968.

McCall, M., M. Lombardo, and A. Morrison. *The Lessons of Experience.* New York: Lexington Books, 1988.

McCluggage, D. *The Centered Skier.* New York: Bantam New Age Books, 1977.

McLuhan, M., and B. Nevitt. *Take Today: The Executive as Dropout.* New York: Harcourt Brace Jovanovich, 1972.

McLuhan, M. *Understanding Media.* Cambridge, Mass.: The MIT Press, 1964.

Moody, R. *Laugh After Laugh.* Jacksonville, Fla.: Headwaters Press, 1978.

Murphy, M. *The Future of the Body.* Los Angeles: Tarcher/Putnam, 1992.

Ornish, D. *Eat More, Weigh Less.* New York: HarperCollins, 1993.

Ornstein, R. *The Evolution of Consciousness.* New York: Prentice-Hall, 1991.

Ornstein, R., and D. Sobel. *The Healing Brain.* New York: Simon and Schuster, 1987.

Ornstein, R., and D. Sobel. *Healthy Pleasures.* Reading, Mass.: Addison Wesley, 1989.

Ornstein, R. *The Psychology of Consciousness.* New York: Penguin, 1972.

Pelletier, K. *Mind as Healer, Mind as Slayer.* New York: Dell Publishing, 1977.

Pelletier, K. *Sound Mind, Sound Body.* New York: Simon and Schuster, 1994.

Peters, T. *The Tom Peters Seminar.* New York: Vintage, 1994.

Pieper, J. *Leisure: the Basis of Culture.* New York: Mentor-Omega, 1963.

Pirsig, R. *Zen and the Art of Motorcycle Maintenance.* New York: Bantam Books, 1974.

Robertson, J., and T. Monte. *Peak-Performance Living.* New York: Harper-Collins, 1996.

Rossi, E. L., and D. Nimmons. *The 20-Minute Break.* Los Angeles: Jeremy Tarcher Inc., 1991.

Rossi, E. L. *The Psychobiology of Mind-Body Healing.* New York: Norton, 1993.

Schor, J. *The Overworked American.* New York: Basic Books, 1991.

Schwartz, T. *What Really Matters.* New York: Bantam, 1995.

Seligman, M. *Learned Optimism.* New York: Pocket Books, 1991.

Selye, H. *Stress Without Distress.* New York: Signet, 1974.

Somer, E. *Food and Mood.* New York: Henry Holt, 1995.

Stack, J. *The Great Game of Business.* New York: Currency Doubleday, 1992.

Suzuki, S. *Zen Mind, Beginner's Mind.* New York: Weatherhill, 1970.

Tarnas, R. *The Passion of the Western Mind.* New York: Ballantine Books, 1991.

Thayer, R. E. *The Origin of Everyday Moods.* New York: Oxford University Press, 1996.

Weil, A. *Natural Health, Natural Medicine.* New York: Houghton Mifflin, 1995.

Weinstein, M. *Managing to Have Fun.* New York: Simon and Schuster, 1996.

Wurtman, J. *Managing Your Mind and Mood Through Food.* New York: Harper & Row, 1986.

ABOUT THE AUTHOR

A poll conducted by the *Journal of Business Strategy* selected Peter McLaughlin, along with Tom Peters and Peter Drucker, as one of the best business speakers in the nation.

Peter is the coauthor of the best-selling book *Mentally Tough: The Principles of Winning at Sports Applied to Winning in Business.* For fifteen years, he has studied the leading research on optimizing health and performance, and has delivered seminars to a Fortune 500 clientele that includes AT&T, American Express, Goldman Sachs, Hewlett Packard, IBM, Marriott, Microsoft, Oracle, PepsiCo, Prudential, and United Artists. Peter's innovative programs have been featured in *USA Today*, *Fast Company* and on CNN, among numerous other newspapers and television programs.

Prior to his work in the peak performance field, Peter pursued a variety of educational and business activities: he received a master's degree in English Literature, he was on the faculty of Regis University in Denver, he owned a wine shop and wrote the wine column for the Rocky Mountain News, and he was president of McLaughlin Company Realtors for ten years. His creative business achievements led the Tarrytown Conference Center in New York to select him as "one of the top 100 most innovative executives in America."

Peter is the president of McLaughlin Company, where he and a team of experts have developed comprehensive, state-of-the-art programs that help businesspeople maximize their health and performance.

For more information on Peter McLaughlin or his programs, visit www.petermclaughlin.com or contact him at peter@petermclaughlin.com.